DOCTORS GET CANCER TOO

DOCTORS GET CANCER TOO

An Hachette UK Company
www.hachette.co.uk

Vie Books, an imprint of Summersdale Publishers Ltd
Part of Octopus Publishing Group Limited
Carmelite House
50 Victoria Embankment
LONDON
EC4Y 0DZ
UK

www.summersdale.com

Printed and bound by CPI Group (UK) Ltd, Croydon, CR0 4YY

ISBN: 978-1-78783-813-0

Substantial discounts on bulk quantities of Summersdale books are available to corporations, professional associations and other organizations. For details contact general enquiries: telephone: +44 (0) 1243 771107 or email: enquiries@summersdale.com.

The author and the publisher cannot accept responsibility for any misuse or misunderstanding of any information contained herein, or any loss, damage or injury, be it health, financial or otherwise, suffered by any individual or group acting upon or relying on information contained herein. None of the views or suggestions in this book is intended to replace medical opinion from a doctor who is familiar with your particular circumstances. If you have concerns about your health, please seek professional advice.

DOCTORS GET CANCER TOO

A DOCTOR'S
DIARY OF LIFE
AND RECOVERY
FROM CANCER

DR PHILIPPA KAYE

For my children, Harrison, Edward and Madeline.
I would fight this or any battle for all eternity in order
to spend even one more day with you.

CONTENTS

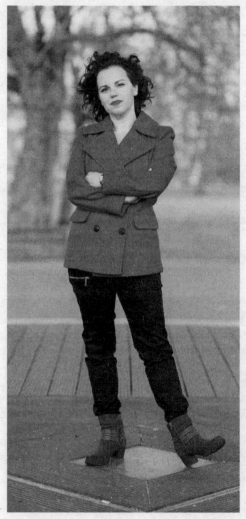

ABOUT THE AUTHOR

Dr Philippa Kaye MBBS (Hons), MA Hons (Cantab), MRCGP (2009), DCH, DRCOG, DFSRH is a GP with a particular interest in children's, women's and sexual health. She has been a GP for over a decade in both the NHS and private sectors. In addition to her general medical and GP qualifications, she holds the Diploma of the Royal College of Obstetrics and Gynaecology, the Diploma of the Faculty of Sexual and Reproductive Healthcare as well as the Diploma of Child Health (from the Royal College of Paediatrics and Child Health). She has written multiple books on women's and children's health, the most recent of which was *The M Word: Everything You Need to Know About the Menopause*, and she regularly contributes to the national press, with a weekly column in *Woman* magazine. She has appeared regularly on *This Morning*, the BBC, Channel 5 and Sky News as well as multiple radio programmes. She is the GP ambassador for Jo's Cervical Cancer Trust. Her days are filled with a mix of general practice, media work and her other job – being a mum! She was diagnosed with colorectal cancer in May 2019.

FOREWORD BY SARA COX

Cancer is a spectre that hangs over us all. We all know someone who's dealing with it; we all fundraise to fight it. We pray we don't get it. We change our lifestyle to minimize the risks. We have smears, we check our boobs and balls. We feel for lumps, praying our search will be fruitless.

But when that search becomes a suspicion and that suspicion becomes a diagnosis, what then? And how do we feel when we put our bodies in the hands of the medical profession?

This is the story of a woman on both sides, a doctor with a cancer diagnosis. A mum, a friend, a daughter and a GP.

Dr Philippa Kaye's book is a frank diary of her cancer journey and explores how it feels when you straddle two worlds, being a doctor and cancer patient. It acknowledges that when it comes to cancer, although knowledge is power, sometimes ignorance is bliss.

INTRODUCTION

Why write a diary and, perhaps even more relevant, why seek to publish something which contains your innermost, deepest thoughts, especially at the darkest moments of your life, when you probably are not your best self?

Out of the blue at the age of thirty-nine I was diagnosed with bowel cancer and, try as I might have done to carry on like nothing had happened, at the time it was nothing short of disastrous, momentous and life-changing. Or so I thought. I was correct in some ways – a cancer diagnosis and treatment are traumatic and sometimes seemingly impossibly difficult – but importantly it does not have to be the beginning of the end. Unfortunately, I have to rely on cliché and hyperbole, as most of us diagnosed with cancer invariably do. That said, if you can't use extremes when faced with a cancer diagnosis, when can you?

I wrote this diary as a kind of catharsis, a sort of emotional vomit on the page, as a way of trying to process and structure the many, often conflicting emotions that cancer brings. These feelings are huge and complex. For me, writing them down, or writing down the order of what was happening to me, was an attempt to contain a situation which was entirely out of my control. To the writer part of me this diary seems really chaotic – so many thoughts, no structure and so much volume! I suppose it reflects the turmoil of my thoughts at that time, so please excuse me when I segue into the next topic with seemingly no connection whatsoever.

To answer the second part of the question, why seek to publish the diary, it took a long time after my diagnosis, many, many days of writing, for the thought to even enter my consciousness. This diary was private, for me and for me alone; no one else read it and even now my husband has not. But as time passed I began to realize that much of what I was writing was about me, being simultaneously a doctor and a patient and the insight that being in both worlds brings. The cancer community, medical or not, is phenomenal, full of support, help and advice. And yet one of the hardest parts about having cancer and treatment is the feeling of isolation that it brings, and I began to realize that by documenting my thoughts (and subsequently publishing them), I could potentially help others feel supported and connected to another person who in some way does not simply sympathize with their experience, but empathizes and truly understands it, having lived it myself. I would be honoured to be that person for you – if reading this makes you feel less alone, or just that someone gets it.

One in two of us will have cancer at some point in our lives, perhaps the most feared diagnosis of all. In the public consciousness, a cancer diagnosis means a death sentence – it means the end, or at least the beginning of the end. But that could not be further from the truth, for many of us, for most of us, cancer is something we are cured of or which we recover from. Even if your cancer cannot be cured, more and more of us are living with cancer for longer than ever, with new treatments and therapies being found.

Many of the cancer diaries out there, wonderful as they are, are published after death. Even as you read them you know what the outcome will be, rather like in *Romeo and Juliet*! They have huge value, however heartbreaking they and the afterwords written by a loved one may be. But this book is not a cancer diary about death, or preparing for death – this is a cancer diary about living, about survival, because that is what most of us who are diagnosed with cancer will do: we survive. Medicine can do wonderful things, but perhaps what cannot be provided by medicine – be it support or understanding, whether you have cancer or not, or are helping someone with cancer – we can give to each other. I hope that this helps you along the way.

WEDNESDAY 8 MAY 2019

Yesterday I was diagnosed with colon cancer.

It is shit.

Literally, I have the shit cancer.

And I saw it myself on the screen.

There are times when being a doctor and a patient is pretty great – when you see your baby's heartbeat on the pregnancy scan, and when you know what you need, what to ask for and who to see. Then there are times when it is pretty crap – when your kids are seriously ill and all you think of are the worst-case scenarios you have witnessed. And times like yesterday, when you look at a screen showing your insides and see something so clearly abnormal that you say: "What is that?"

I should probably backtrack a bit; no one just ends up on a couch hugging their knees with a tube up their bum without a bit of backstory. Though some people may well enjoy that sort of thing.

Since the birth of my youngest, my daughter, four years ago, I've been having some intermittent pain in my pelvis. I've had multiple pelvic surgeries, including three Caesarean sections, and the removal of my appendix and an ectopic pregnancy. I presumed that the pain was linked to some scar tissue and didn't think much of it. I am like that, and I think many of us are – if we can explain something, or if it isn't bothering us, we put it out of our minds and keep going.

But in the past three or four months the pain has got worse, so eventually I saw a doctor who I used to work with when I was a junior doctor. He also delivered my first baby. Although you would have thought that having him examine me would be weird, it really isn't – doctors don't think about that sort of thing, they just get on with the examination. The ultrasound seemed normal, but I was referred to a colorectal surgeon – one who I refer patients to regularly – to check out my bowel, just to be sure there was nothing there before considering surgery. The surgeon thought everything was fine, but advised me to have an MRI (magnetic resonance imaging scan), as it was better for seeing scar tissue or other problems.

The MRI showed up a very slight abnormality, a small bit of spasm in the lower colon. This could have been anything and nothing, and while most radiologists wouldn't have commented on it, this one advised the surgeon to perform a colonoscopy, even though the surgeon was confident the results would come back normal.

A word of caution to anyone who may have to have a colonoscopy: bowel prep is revolting. Before the procedure, the patient must drink a laxative to help completely clear the bowel of waste. My drink was like peach-flavoured seawater and made me feel unbearably sick all day. Not much happened for five hours, which was somewhat surprising, and even after the second dose when I did start hosing Armageddon from my behind I was still surprised as I thought there would be much more.

There I was, waiting for the colonoscopy. I became irritated because bowel prep isn't the most fun and I knew the results were going to be normal – and therefore a waste of time – and I would have to have exploratory surgery to remove scar tissue anyway. The surgeon breezed in, said he thought it would be fine, as I suspected, but there was a 1 per cent chance at my age of having a polyp so big it couldn't be removed via the scope.

Bowel cancers grow from polyps, which are initially benign before turning cancerous. A benign polyp can be removed during colonoscopy, and even a small cancerous polyp could be removed that way without the need for surgery. With all cancers, the earlier you are diagnosed, the easier they are to treat and the more likely you are to have a better prognosis. So, the earlier the better.

The outfit provided for the colonoscopy was simply sublime. You could wear it to the Met Gala and quite frankly no one would raise an eyebrow. Dark blue "modesty shorts", though nothing modest there as they have a great gaping hole in the back for arse access. Then the routine went as follows: cannula in, bit of sedation, lie on your left side, tube up the bum and off we go. Only I don't think the sedation really did much as I remember every single moment of what came next. Within seconds we saw something.

Me: "What is that?"

Surgeon: "Erm, that is unusual. There seems to be a growth." Pause. "I think you are going to need an operation."

As he tried to move the scope past the lesion it hurt, but I told him I would manage and to keep going.

"No," he said, "it is hurting you, and I don't need to hurt you."

That is when I realized that I was going for surgery. He was going to hurt me plenty then, so he didn't need to hurt me now.

I knew and he knew I knew it was cancer. And the softer and kinder the nurses in the room became, the more certain I was. The surgeon was caring and reassuring and kept up the gentle constant patter. All the while he was talking, he took lots of biopsies, small samples of tissue to be examined by pathologists using a microscope, that will tell us exactly what we are dealing with.

To complete the ordeal, the surgeon gave me my first tattoo, at the age of thirty-nine and a half, albeit an internal tattoo on my bowel, so he would know exactly where to make the incision during surgery. The tattooing stung a bit but then I think getting any tattoo does. All I could think was that my mum would not be impressed as she doesn't like tattoos!

Once the scope had been completed, I was wheeled back to a cubicle and the doctor said he'd be with me shortly, asking if I had anyone with me. I had sent my husband, Ben, to work, as we didn't think anything would show up, but my mum had driven to the hospital to bring me home again. He asked if I wanted her.

Doctors and nurses are taught how to deliver bad news, and it starts by going to a quiet separate room, and encouraging the patient to have a loved one with them. It was these actions as well as their words, which I know so very well from the other side, that made it worse, so much worse, because I knew, I knew I was in trouble, I knew it was cancer. Perhaps many of us do – all those episodes of *ER* or *Casualty* pay off!

My mum took one look at me and asked what it was. I told her that I had colorectal cancer. I am not sure it is supposed to happen like that.

The surgeon arrived: "Philippa, as you know, we saw a growth, an unusual growth."

And then I did what we expect patients to do. You see, doctors don't say that they have bad news and follow it with the C word. Instead they say something like "You know we did the test because we were looking for something, and we found something", to which the patient asks the doctor if they found cancer. This way the patient comes to their own realization that it is cancer.

Without even really thinking about it, I duly replied, "It is cancer, right, so let's use the word."

"Yes, it is cancer," the surgeon replied, "but you will be fine."

I don't really remember too much of what came next and writing it down here feels blurry. He showed me where the scars would be, told me I would be in hospital for seven to ten days. He told me where the cancer was in relation to the rectum and that there was around a 10 per cent chance that I would need a stoma, a temporary ileostomy, a bag from your tummy which connects to your bowel and collects your poo instead of it going out of your bottom. He reassured me that 10 per cent is small.

"I had a one per cent chance of finding a polyp at my age and that was smaller," I replied.

"Well, yes," he replied.

◆

I was then sent for a CT (computed tomography) chest, a scan to look for spread, and a CT pneumocolon, which is a virtual colonoscopy, and something you do for people who aren't able to have a colonoscopy or in this situation when you can't get past something.

The radiographer asked me how I was. I replied that I had just been told I have colorectal cancer and couldn't stop a tear creeping out. She was lovely but literally ran away to get the trappings of grief, a glass of water, some tissues – she needed to keep busy, to do something. More tubes in the bum for the CT pneumocolon: this time my bowel was puffed up with air and then an injection of a medical dye (called contrast) which helps doctors interpret the scans. I had been warned about the side effects, and indeed had discussed them with patients, though not everyone gets them. Within seconds, I noticed a metallic taste in my mouth and then the sensation of heat in my genitals as if you have wet yourself, though you have not.

Tummy bloated with air, half naked in the changing room, mum waiting in the waiting room, I rang my best friend, a child psychotherapist, and asked her what to tell my children. I told her I needed her to be professional, to just tell me and not react. Within me I felt my personal, professional wall have a few more bricks added to it.

All doctors have to have a wall. It protects us, our souls, our hearts. Sometimes people say it makes us hard, but it doesn't; we can still be empathetic and sympathetic while the wall is up. Occasionally patients make chinks in the wall – though it happens less the more experienced you become – and when they do, you recognize them, are human for a bit and then have to move on.

Doctors are thrown into a world of grief and rage, death and unfairness at a relatively young age. I was twenty-four and exposed to dead people and grieving families on a daily basis. I have seen kids and babies die, I have seen people hurt each other in the worst ways possible, and I have seen loneliness and pain. If I let all of that in I would drown.

So my wall went up. I think it is still up, it protects me right now, it means that I don't have to think about anything, about the ramifications of being told I have cancer, that I don't let it in, I just keep going, be that telling my husband, telling my children, doing bath time with them, or reading or bedtime. My wall means that I can keep functioning right now.

◆

The children are four, seven and eleven.

Their responses:

The four-year-old: who will take me to school? Totally age-appropriate response.

The seven-year-old: came straight over to give me a massive hug and then recoiled almost instantly. "You can't catch cancer, can you?" he said as he backed rapidly away! Followed by "What if X doesn't work, what if Y doesn't work? What if you… ?" (Here he drew his hand across his neck as if cutting his head off.)

The eleven-year-old: wanted to talk about a character in the book he was reading who has gastric cancer and will die.

And then they went to bed. We watched TV and I waited for the surgeon to phone with the results of the scan. Time dragged on, 10 p.m.… 10.30 p.m.… Emotionally exhausted, I went to bed. He rang at 10.38 p.m. The scan showed no spread, and I took a breath – I think the first proper breath I had taken since 3 p.m. – and determinedly went to sleep.

Sleep is one of the first things you lose in times of psychological stress, and sure as damn it I was up from 5 a.m. and couldn't switch off my thoughts.

There is nothing to do today. I need to tell some people and make plans. Thankfully I was not due at surgery today; I had set it aside for writing copy for the magazines and websites I write for.

Nothing will change until I see the surgeon in two days and then have the op. And yet I can't concentrate. I told the kids' school, so the teachers would be prepared if they have questions, and I told the parents of their closest friends in case they told them, all by message as I can't deal with their reactions – even reading them by text is exhausting. I told myself I could just carry on as normal for the next week until the surgery, but I haven't been able to write a word of copy. Instead I write this.

THURSDAY 9 MAY

Today I went to work. Perhaps this is surprising, that I would want to go to work, but it feels like nothing has happened as yet and I knew I would be able to lose myself in clinic, that working would be a good distraction.

Middlest child asked me if I was frightened today. I said that I was frightened, frightened of being in pain, because I am, but that the doctors will give me medicine to make the pain go away. He seemed content with that. Was it the truth? Partly. I did not lie to him, I won't lie to them to protect them, but perhaps telling some of the truth, leaving parts out, helps us all. I am frightened of the pain, but in general I'm afraid of so much more, more than perhaps I can even verbalize to myself right now.

Telling people is the worst. Although it isn't a secret or something shameful to be hidden, it is private, and I can't bear the thought of a gaggle of women at the school gates wanting to talk about it. But my life is busy and complicated and there are lots of people who need to know. My work; the receptionists at my private practice; my agent, as the first edit of my next book is due to arrive next week; the chair of the board of school governors where I am vice chair; the friends we are due to have for lunch next weekend. And then I need to start making plans for the kids – who'll be able to take them to ballet or Scouts, etc. This involves asking for favours, which I don't find easy, so I feel I need to tell them too.

It is exhausting. Because they all have a reaction. Which is fine, and understandable, but their reaction is about them and I can't handle any more people's emotions. I've got a grip on me currently – my wall is up about 3 metres higher than usual – and denial, while not always a healthy coping mechanism, can be useful for survival. Think about the next step, don't consider what might come after and just keep going. I have my kids' emotions to deal with, worry about and protect. My husband's, my parents' and siblings', who are all great but I know they are upset and that their tears are about me. I feel guilty for hurting them, for putting all of them through this trauma. It isn't my fault and yet I feel guilty, and a bit embarrassed, embarrassed of the attention, embarrassed of the eyes looking at me, at knowing everyone would be talking about me (even if in a kind, concerned way).

It is all very conflicting – I seem to want the best of both worlds here. I am embarrassed by the attention but also want to be nurtured and looked after, and then I feel guilty for not even knowing what I want, or wanting too many opposing things. I want people to show me that they care about me by ringing, but I also don't want to answer, don't want to speak to them and I don't want to have to rehash over and over and over how we got here and what might happen next. I want them to message and I might message back, but if they don't I will be upset and cross! Spoilt? Me? Never! But maybe I'm not spoilt, but conflicted; feelings, especially big, huge feelings like this, are complex!

In a nutshell, outside of my inner circle that I need to protect, which I suppose includes me, I can't deal with your shock and grief. I am not sure I am dealing with mine, maybe not even acknowledging it, so I sure as hell can't handle yours. Perhaps that is the conflict: I want to be nurtured, to be reassured, but your reaction is about you, not me.

FRIDAY 10 MAY

I went to bed last night and fell asleep pretty quickly but was up from 2.30 to about 5 a.m. The world is a dark, lonely place then. I know my insomnia was anxiety about today's appointments but knowing the reason doesn't make it disappear. When I woke up at 2.30 a.m. it was from a dream about conjunctivitis and my eyes were stinging. When I brought my hand to my eyes they, and my cheeks, were wet. I must have been crying in my sleep.

My husband and I set off to the train station, rather like we were going on a slightly bizarre date! We spent almost an hour with the consultant. Doctors always say to patients, bring someone else, you won't remember it all, and write down your questions beforehand, otherwise as soon as you leave you will remember something else. So, being a good patient, I wrote them down, literally twenty questions!

We went through them and quite frankly it was a lot to take in. It's no wonder people forget.

Notes from the consultation:

- It *is* the colon cancer we think it is, that I was told it is. I need a partial colectomy, where part of the colon is removed.
- It is 15 centimetres above the anus and, from a surgical point of view, it is just on the cusp of being risky as they cut 5 centimetres below the mass (which is about 5 centimetres itself) and then take away lots of bowel above. When the anastomosis (the join) is within 15 centimetres of the anus there is a 10–17 per cent chance it will break down. If it does it will be really painful and requires a second, emergency surgery to create a stoma. 15 minus 5 centimetres is 10 centimetres from the anus but the doctor thinks he could manage it. A 10–17 per cent chance of having an ileostomy, a stoma, a bag... temporary but still.
- Two consultant colorectal surgeons will be operating, along with one urological consultant as I may need a ureteric stent due to a 10 per cent risk of ureteric injury – basically a straw in the tube which connects the kidney to the bladder, in order to protect it. The doctor says that this stent will hurt, hurt so much I will think the anastomosis (the join in my bowel) is leaking, but he will know the difference.
- The surgery is going to be long, about six–eight hours.

- I'll spend one night in ICU, with a catheter, venous access for lots of drips and fluids, oxygen, patient-controlled morphine for painkillers and maybe a nasogastric tube, a tube that goes from your nose to your stomach to suck out your stomach juices if needed. (I remember practising putting them in each other as a medical student; everyone was gagging – it was pretty horrid.)

- Bowel prep before the surgery – again! (The prep was so painful and I was so nauseous the first time round, as I have a partial obstruction, a blockage in my bowel, and there is simply not enough room in there for everything to pass through! Not looking forward to it again but it makes sense to need a clean bowel, so there's less risk of infection.)

- The bowel rest afterwards – day one: 30 millilitres fluid per hour; day two: 60 millilitres per hour; day three: 90 millilitres per hour; day four: 120 millilitres and a sip of chicken soup (I don't even bloody like soup, especially chicken soup – the only Jew who doesn't!).

- On about day five apparently I will pass gas. The gas expands in the area and the surgeon reports there is excruciating pain for 20 minutes or so. As soon as a fart is released the worst is over.

- After about seven–ten days in hospital I should be ready to go home, going from a liquid-only diet to purée, then soft food. (I thought my days of making baby food were done!)

- Potentially my lifelong constipation will be over! On the other hand, my anus may forget the difference between gas, liquid and air – anuses really are very clever, but there may be a time, or indeed forever, when you cannot risk a fart! There could be diarrhoea (anything from twice a day to twenty times) or no diarrhoea, or constipation, or no change at all; who knows what the future will hold for my bowel habits!

The surgeon mentioned pain a lot during our consultation, which made me nervous. Usually we talk about pain post-operatively and about how we will make sure you are pain-free, and it isn't that we disregard the suffering but perhaps we downplay it, as a patient's mindset is hugely important pre-operation. Thinking you are going to come out the other side fine and pain-free leads to better recovery. So when a doctor says things like "excruciating pain", or "hurt so much you will think it is breaking down", there is nothing to expect but agony and it is really quite terrifying.

Pain aside, some parts of the briefing sounded like plumbing, which essentially it is. Disconnect the pipes, take out the rotten bit and join the pipes back up. But it was when he said that he cuts the blood supply and then rejoins it, followed by a quick tea break for thirty minutes before coming back and seeing if it all looks vascular and pink instead of blue that he really sounded like our plumber – do a bit of this, stop for a cuppa, do a bit more… Good surgeons know that what they do is only part of the picture. The impact on you as a patient and your recovery can be far more significant than the procedure itself.

◆

Later, on the Radio 4 afternoon show, I talked about cancer screening programmes, including bowel screenings. Oh, the irony, talking about low uptake numbers, when I am over two decades too young for the bowel-screening programme (which at the time of writing starts at age sixty and involves a poo test) in the first place!

SATURDAY 11 MAY

T-minus four days to op day.

I think I had a panic attack last night, a sense of rising panic and impending doom – chest tight, short of breath, shaking. A sense of terror about what is happening. This whole process can't be good for your heart! The cancer is the last thing I think of before I go to sleep, the first thing that enters my head when I wake up. It is all-encompassing and seems insurmountable, a veritable, personal Everest that is looming over and controlling everything.

Today we went to the aquarium with the kids, a place I normally find rather peaceful with huge tanks of slowly undulating rays and sharks. I wept my way around. Moments of solitude and quiet are overwhelming.

Later I thought I would rest for an hour. Except I didn't. Instead I wrote my "just in case" letters, to my parents, Ben, my children. Just in case something happens to me, just in case I don't come home. I don't think this is going to happen, I really don't, but I am scared of the pain, scared of what follows. I am also terrified of dying from this, but not frightened that I will die on the table. Still, I wrote them just in case.

How do you write letters to those you love most in the world in case you die? Where do you start? How can you end? Do you give advice, make requests, declare undying love? Of course you declare undying love, but the rest? If I knew that I was dying maybe I would write birthday cards, wedding cards, but these are letters just in case. I wept and wept while writing them, hot, burning tears streaming down my face, crying silently as I didn't want anyone to hear. I cried so much that I have felt ill all afternoon with puffy, burning eyes and a headache. Yet I still haven't told my husband I wrote the letters, for fear of being not laughed at exactly but pooh-poohed, because for him the idea that I might not wake up is simply not possible. He won't let it in.

Today is not a good day.

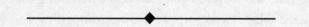

There is a doctors' support group I am a member of, and venting to them has been useful, perhaps because they understand the fear of the doctor-patient, or perhaps because they are just good people. There was a ring on the doorbell and a package arrived from them, containing such thoughtful gifts: dry-mouth anti-nausea sweets, dry shampoo, lip balm, eye mask, hand cream, smoothie pouches to freeze for when I'm on my liquid diet and wet wipes for the inevitable sore bum when it starts to work again. Essentially it was a care package from those used to dealing with the sick and hospitalized, a hospital survival kit. Such care, such thoughtfulness.

Are cancer gifts a thing then? Apart from the fantastic gift of cancer of course, do I get cancer gifts? Are there such things as *Sorry you have cancer. Sorry it is up your bum* cards? Maybe there is a business here: sorry you have bowel cancer – have some wet wipes for your bum; sorry you have breast cancer – here is a one-sided padded bra; sorry you have cervical cancer – here are some sanitary towels; sorry you have prostate cancer – here is some Viagra. There is a gap in the market! Perhaps I have found a bonus to cancer – you get "Sorry you have cancer" gifts.

In my community anything and everything is made better or celebrated with food. Had a baby? I'm making food. Someone dies? I'm making food. Got a new job? I'm making food. What will my loved ones do when they can't bring me food? There is a need to do, to bring, to feel that you have contributed in some way, and without food that is going to be hard.

◆

At home I am surrounded by love, support, messages to bolster me, gifts, offers of help of the practical and psychological kind. People are here for me, and I know this. And yet I am entirely alone. No one else is doing this but me. I was alone at the scope, alone at the CT and although Ben was with me at the consultation I was still alone. I will go down to the operating theatre surrounded by nurses, porters and doctors but I will be alone. I will be looked after by a myriad of healthcare professionals afterwards, but I will be alone. I am happy in my own company, but I don't like being alone.

SUNDAY 12 MAY

T-minus three days to op day.

The rumour mill was churning so I decided to send a WhatsApp message to the groups for each of my children's classes. I said that no one needed to message or phone and actually I meant that, but I was utterly unprepared for the barrage of good wishes, feeling and love that came my way. So many messages, voice messages, texts offering help, prayers, rotas for school and food. It feels like charity, and I am not sure that I want it, or need it to be honest. I politely declined the majority but said that I may need help with the school rota, etc., as I don't know when I will be able to do the school run. Right now I am a hot topic of gossip but will the offers of help still be there six months down the line if I have to have chemo and could be out of action for a while? Wow, that is bitchy, isn't it? Why can't I just accept what is being offered? But having essentially dedicated my life and career choices to helping others, it is hard to be on the receiving end, to ask for and accept help.

Today I started planning. You never would have guessed that I am slightly controlling from my pages of notes! I write a plan for every day I'm at the hospital, from who is picking up who from where, to what is for each meal. I won't even know if they stick to it and it wouldn't matter if they ate fish fingers for the next week, but it helps me to feel that I have some control when everything internally is utterly out of my hands. The stages of treatment for the cancer are careering along like an unstoppable juggernaut with me being strapped in for a not very fun ride.

My lists include when to do the laundry, to leave money for the piano teacher and to plan a Tesco order. But what I am actually saying is: I am still here, I am still with you, I am still your mother, your wife, I am still looking after you, I am doing my best to keep everything as normal as it can be, I love you, I love you, I love you.

MONDAY 13 MAY

T-minus two days to op day.

My mum and I have always gone baby shopping together. We scouted buggies, cots and clothes, post-maternity paper pants, nipple pads and more. Today we went cancer shopping. I knew I would need soft bras and big pants after surgery – soft bras because my tummy would be filled with gas, which takes some time to go down, so wires may be uncomfortable, and big pants to ensure the line of the knickers isn't in the same place as my new wound – as well as other soft things, from soft fluffy socks, and soft hair bobbles and hairbands (even a hair bobble can hurt lying on your back), to soft and bigger elasticated-waist PJs. Soft, soft, like for a baby, so nothing irritates you when you are already in pain. My clothes are generally quite fitted so we went to get some looser tops and if anyone was following us around the shops, heard our conversations and witnessed our slightly hysterical laughter, they would have thought we were insane! All the tops had slogans on them like "Living my best life", so we would create new versions appropriate for me:

- Living my best life… with/without cancer.
- This is me… with/without cancer.
- Thank you. Next!… Thank you, cancer. Next!

Our shopping trip included buying bits for the kids when I am away: mini chocolate treats for breakfast (they will really know I miss them if they are allowed them), a comic each, some stickers and more. Tomorrow I will wrap the gifts, and write cards for each child for the few days when I am in the hospital. These are little things, but for me, at this moment, they are heavy with meaning. It might be a little treat which they will inhale and probably not think of moments later, but I am trying to say that although I am away, I am still here, I am your mother, I love you. And perhaps even more weighty: don't forget about me.

Later on in the afternoon, I picked up the kids from school. Now all the parents know, waiting in the playground is like running a gauntlet! I could see lots of them nudging each other and whispering, some sympathetic looks. Some people came and gave me a pat before walking away silently (what is that?!), some people came over and then – quite clearly remembering – swerved away with a guilty glance, others clearly wanted to talk, or to hear the news. Instead of dealing with all of them, I accosted two actual friends and busied myself talking to them; it seemed to put off some of the circling!

◆

My final thought of the day was what would you have for your last meal? Perhaps a dinner party question but it suddenly had more weight! Previously I would have said sushi, or duck and pancakes, but tonight I turn to comfort, to a childhood school holiday treat of breaded chicken (in a ring shape) and pasta drowned in ketchup – not healthy, not sophisticated, but comforting. From tomorrow I start my bowel prep and then it will be days before I eat again.

TUESDAY 14 MAY

T-minus one day to op day.

I slapped the warpaint on this morning for a media meeting, a bright breezy Instagram story, detailing my morning of meetings and a stroll through Borough Market, and a serious video post for my followers, all before coming home for bowel prep. The contrast between the projected normality of my morning and the turmoil of my mind felt bizarre and is a great example of "Insta reality" vs actual reality!

I barely sleep any more. The world is not a kind place in the middle of the night; it is lonely and cold and your darkest thoughts come to the fore and play over and over.

First bowel prep pint in – that stuff makes me feel so, so sick. To distract myself I wrote cards for the first five days when I am away, until the kids can see me again, just little bits of nonsense chatter really. Then to pack for the worst holiday ever, but at least I didn't have to decide how many pairs of shoes or sandals to take, just fluffy socks and slippers!

All of this then led me on to the second pint of bowel prep, which I quite simply could not get or keep down. I was retching, bringing up each mouthful no matter how slowly I went. In desperation I messaged the surgeon, who advised me to keep trying, to keep sipping after a break but that he will manage the surgery come what may. In medical school we were taught that "the solution to the pollution is in the dilution". In other words, if there is stool in the surgical field where you operate, wash and wash and wash it away. After all, we carry out bowel surgery in an emergency, where no one has taken bowel prep! Still, I feel that I should be giving myself the best chance; although you can't clean the bacteria out of your gut, not having a shit-filled bowel would be desirable and I don't seem to be able to do that. It feels like I am failing already.

I keep trying to run through what it would be like waking up with a bag, so that if it is there it doesn't come as a crashing disappointment. But each time I think about it in my head and imagine waking up to find it is there it upsets me so, so much that I don't seem to be able to imagine life with it. I know I would survive it, I know many people manage, but it is daunting. I don't know how to prepare myself for it, to not be disappointed by it. Perhaps I cannot. Like most women I have had some qualms about my body, bits I like better than others, and bits I am not so fond of. Now my relationship with my body and how it looks is changing again. My body is currently housing a cancer, and it feels like that cancer is out to get me. It has sort of become personified, at least in my head, as something plotting malevolently away inside me. Why is my body out to get me? I look after it, I don't smoke, I exercise, I eat well, I am doing it right and yet my body is coming after me, or at least some part of my bowel is. I know this is a feeling and not a fact, that it is the cancer, not me. That it came from my body but it isn't me, and by me I mean the essence of who I am. The cancer is not me. I need to learn to disassociate this cancer from me; I hope that removing the cancer will help.

◆

The eldest was upset tonight, sobbing and sobbing. He doesn't want things to change, he is frightened they will find something they can't fight. He cried and I cried along, and then vomited from the prep and then went back and cried together some more. I told him that I will still be here and even when he doesn't see me for a few days I am still here, and in his heart and in his brain.

Kissing your kids goodnight when you won't see them for a while, and not because you are being whisked off on a romantic getaway, or even for work, is a delicate process. There is the urge to prolong – one more hug, one more kiss – almost as if I have turned into the three-year-old not wanting to go to nursery, as if I am the child and not them! Instead, a hug and a kiss and words of love without tears, helped by the fact that the middlest and eldest started arguing about something entirely inconsequential (nothing out of the ordinary there) which puts me in my place and then all three children are in bed.

I asked the surgeon for one sleeping pill for tonight. I am not pro sleepers at all – they are addictive and stop working within weeks, meaning you need more and more – but I don't think I can take being up all night, especially as I have to be in at 6 a.m. He prescribed without hesitation.

Nothing left to do now. I have prepared as much as I can – prepared for myself, prepared for my family in every practical way I can think of and hopefully in some psychological ways too. Tomorrow it and I will be in someone else's hands. See you on the other side.

WEDNESDAY 15 MAY

Written in retrospect on Monday 20 May

T-minus zero days.

Op day.

Written in retrospect, days later than I expected as I thought I would be well enough to write almost straight away, yet probably a day or so too early as sitting up and writing is a huge effort, physically, mentally and psychologically.

Sitting in a chair in ICU.

Once at the hospital, I was checked in, weighed and measured and a cannula inserted. When you go to hospital for surgery you have to tell your story to every healthcare professional, to each nurse and doctor, so you answer the same questions over and over and very, very slowly, time ticks forward.

The consultant anaesthetist came, took my history and told me the plan regarding the anaesthetic, the drugs he would use for sleep, and the ones for pain – a normal cannula for a drip which can contain pain relief, then an epidural and then a spinal anaesthetic, which go into your spine and will be used for pain relief, like the ones you might have when you are having a baby. All this will be done while I'm awake so he can see the level of the anaesthetic block, so he can test where I have sensation and where I do not. And only after all of that prodding and poking, and lying still while they insert all these lines, will there be the anaesthetic gas and sleep. He warned me what else there would be attached to me when I woke up: lots more intravenous lines, an arterial line (drips normally go into veins – this one will go into an artery), maybe a central line which is a huge line for drips and medications which is inserted into some of the largest blood vessels in your body through your neck, and maybe a nasogastric tube. Yet more maybes. I am likely to wake up with a PCA (a patient-controlled analgesia) where you press a button when you need pain relief, which is then delivered through a drip. Maybe, maybe, maybe.

It was so much to take in, from getting a cancer diagnosis to being showered in information and leaflets up to your neck. Knowing the medical terminology and understanding of what each of those things are probably helped the anaesthetist speed up his talk, without having to explain each process, and I suppose it meant that I had less to absorb. I was utterly overwhelmed; how would a non-medic feel?

The surgeon appeared and suddenly it was time to go. My mum was allowed to walk me down, as Ben was at home with the kids to keep things normal for them. The surgeon gave the exact level of confidence you need. Bright and breezy, he had checked the equipment, run through the op with colleagues, etc. I totally felt he had me – I just wasn't sure that I had me! The consultant urologist popped into the anaesthetic room and then it was time for my mum to say goodbye. They said she could maybe stay for the epidural but for me it was time for her to go. We hugged and I cried and she told me to let it all out but I couldn't – it was time to put the game face on, time to go, be brave, bring it on. I cannot imagine how she felt at that point.

So there I was, long white compression stockings on, yellow no-slip socks on top, paper disposable pants and a hospital gown, surrounded by people but alone. You are alone in your head with your thoughts, your mind, alone in your body, in your very soul, and you give all of these, your whole self, to strangers to hold, to protect, to heal, to cure.

———————————◆———————————

Step one – drip placed in your hand.

Step two – curl up in a ball for the epidural. Local anaesthetic works to numb an area, but it burns like a bee sting when it is injected into you – having it injected into your spine is not a nice experience.

Step three – stay curled up while the epidural is placed. The anaesthetist kept up a constant patter, the often meaningless distracting small talk, while at the same time explaining what they are doing, rather like a hairdresser. But this version somehow seemed to include "Just left my needle in your spine there – don't move, don't want to paralyze you, ha ha!"

As the epidural started to work there was a sense of wooziness and light-headedness as my blood pressure fell (which is a normal reaction), so a shot of adrenaline, and whoosh I am back.

Step four – finally on my back and the anaesthetist asks for midazolam, which is a sedative, or what he calls "gin and tonic".

Step five – breathe in the sweet smelling gas (which is the anaesthetic) and the last thing I heard was the anaesthetist say "I've got you"…

———————————◆———————————

A sense of swimming, dragging myself back up to the surface, but not in a gentle way from sleep, rather desperately searching, reaching for air. I can hear someone talking but can't catch what they are saying. Gagging, trying to take a breath and getting nothing. Try again, gasping, can't breathe, and on that second attempt I hear "tube coming out" and there is a rush of sweet air, followed by an intense crushing pain in my chest and shoulders. Gagging, retching, vomiting and being surrounded by people catching vomit, giving meds. And through the pain and nausea one question as I pat my tummy: bag? Bag? No bag. A fleeting sense of elation. Then just pain and nausea. As I come round further and they get these feelings more under control, I become more aware of what is on me: cardiac monitors, oxygen mask, big line in hand, in forearm, arterial line in wrist and yet still not enough access – the anaesthetist puts in more lines. Crushing pain, a heavy weight in the shoulders and chest from the gas of the op and a searing pain in my abdomen.

Surgeon comes in, and I have to check again: "Bag?"

"No bag."

"Did you get it?"

"I took lots out. I think I've got it."

Fleeting sense of elation returns. It passes in seconds – I try to hang on to it.

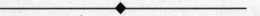

Up on ICU I have no sensation beneath my breasts, so nothing really hurts, but as the night wears on I begin to get a sensation in my right side and press the epidural button continually – it delivers fentanyl, an opiate painkiller. This initial lack of sensation proves to be falsely reassuring.

Not sure I remember much more.

THURSDAY 16 MAY

Written in retrospect on Monday 20 May

This day was a haze of pain.

My right side was agony but I couldn't move my left at all, which was totally numb from breast down. This was the epidural anaesthetic, and the tube in my spine had probably dislodged, meaning one side was numb and the other not. But not only was I numb on one side – I also couldn't move it. The surgeon said to try to get up, and indeed I know that mobilizing is hugely important to recovery, but it was literally an impossibility.

My kids had asked previously how I would wash and I glibly said "bed bath". A bed bath is both a delight and a torture. Agony of being rolled by two nurses followed by the bliss of being cleaned with warm wipes and having cream rubbed into sore skin. Then repeat until they get to your bottom and vulva. I am thirty-nine years old and I do not remember the last time someone wiped my bum for me. I hope to never again. They are soft, they are gentle, they mutter kind words of reassurance and even nonsense aimed to comfort. Even knowing that when I do my job I think of nothing but doing the best job I can, that I don't judge and am not embarrassed, I still feel embarrassed as a patient myself. There is no dignity here.

Wave after wave of pain. Pressing the button over and over, and the meds seemed to deliver unconsciousness for a second or two, but then back into a wave of pain. The cannulas kept blowing, meaning that the drips could not work and they couldn't put more in. My veins are pretty rubbish, so getting a new line in became an insurmountable task. If I lay completely still and no one touched me I could just about manage but anything else was torture. Pain, then button push then descend into nothingness for a glorious few seconds then back up into a screaming blaze of pain.

It was decided I needed a PICC line. This is a long line with two ports which is used when you don't have any veins left. The procedure cannot be done in ICU. Instead it is done by a radiologist and involved being rolled on to a bed, wheeled over the tiny painful bumps, for example of the lift and doorways, then rolled on to the procedure bed, then off, and repeat the process back to ICU. Injecting the bee-stinging local anaesthetic and the pushing or pressure sensation of putting the line in was the least painful part of the process; just stop moving me! The radiologist said a PICC line could last for six months – six months? Six months! I am getting out of here in a week, aren't I? A mantra appeared in my head: this is temporary, it is all just for now, just for now.

Back in ICU and wave after wave of torrents of pain are still present; time merges and blurs until the doctors decide to change the painkillers in the epidural and the patient-controlled analgesia, and suddenly I am there. Me, in pain but not ruled by it, conscious, and not drifting in and out of oblivion. In pain, sure, but in focus of something that I can see

I can win against, the tsunami of pain reduced to an ordinarily stormy sea.

Brushing my teeth that night felt like a HIIT session. As knackering but without the elation of endorphin release. Brushing your teeth is something ordinary, routine, before bed and sleep, but for me it was another night of no sleep. I can't sleep on my back normally, never mind with an immobile leg from the epidural and in pain. Instead I drift in and out. Time passes slowly on ICU; days and nights blur into one – one long, long, long time.

FRIDAY 17 MAY

Written in retrospect on Tuesday 21 May

The plan for the day used to be written on a board by your bed in hospital. It isn't now, in the same way that there is not a board with the names of all the patients and which bed they are in, to protect your confidentiality. My board would have said, *Mobilize* – I have to get up today. It also would have said, *60 mls/hour*; yesterday I had to drink 30 millilitres of water per hour. Who knew 60 millilitres of water was so much? Four tablespoons, two fluid ounces. I burp my way through it slowly, feeling nauseated but I manage, just about, though it takes a surprisingly long time to sip. Before I know it an hour has passed and it is time to start again.

You are all tied up in ICU, literally tied to the bed, not with cuffs or restraints but with wires and lines. Five chest leads (sometimes twelve) which monitor your heart rate and rhythm, oxygen mask or nasal prongs, lines for fluids, for the PCA or other infusions such as antibiotics, a catheter, a blood pressure cuff and weird things attached to your calves to squeeze them intermittently to prevent blood clots.

Time to stand up. I thought I knew what to expect here – I had had Caesarean sections, I had had other surgery, I had seen so many patients through surgery. I thought that I would know what it felt like and what to do. I had no clue. None at all. Getting up after a big surgery, and especially after lying down for forty-eight hours, is not as simple as standing up, or even as simple as standing up slowly; it is a humongous effort as your body remembers what it is like to be upright, and it really doesn't like it. It is normal for this to be tough, for you to need the assistance of a nurse and the physio, and for it to be exhausting, but I had no idea how tough it was going to be. My epidural had been removed and I had to lie flat for an hour, to try to stop an epidural leak developing, which would lead to a severe headache, but after that the bed was raised so I am sitting up. The plan is then to sit up more, scoot your legs over to the side and stand up. Or not. I simply can't get past the legs over the side bit with my body still leaning on the bed. I cannot. The world is spinning, then I see black stars. It simply is not happening, and I am trying, I really am, I want to get up. I am frightened – what happens if I can't? But I can't. I lie back down again and the physio says she will return. Perhaps trying after the hour of completely lying flat was too much. It feels like an enormous failure; it is just standing up, for crying out loud. I didn't even need to stand there long, just simply stand and then sit in the chair, and even that was insurmountable. During recovery it feels like every little failure has a huge negative effect on your psyche, which has a tendency to spiral downward; it is a constant effort to keep going, in all ways.

Ninety minutes later and here we go again. I am getting up come what may. Come what may really wants to come but twenty minutes of sitting supported in bed, then five on the side of the bed and I am upright. Just about upright, with my world spinning, and when the physio asks me to look up I literally see her move over and over again. She asks if the room is spinning or if I am dizzy and I lie and say it wasn't; I wasn't failing again. I don't recommend lying to your care team. I have since told her that I lied that day and am pretty sure she knew but I couldn't not get up again. I had to win this time, I had to get up. Sheer stubbornness won the day and after a few minutes the spinning abated a bit. Two paces later and we are in the chair. This whole excursion to the chair lasted about twenty minutes, most of which was being tied back to the wires and then being untied again, and I am back in bed, exhausted. That night I brush my teeth again. These two activities have taken on marathon proportions.

———————◆———————

I am waiting for the predicted "agonizing pain" before passing wind. My tummy is making such loud, grumbling noises I keep asking if other people can hear them! If you have ever had a tummy bug, or even in general sometimes, you can feel your intestines working; your tummy often rumbles or growls but sometimes you can feel your large intestines moving things along. The gut is lined with smooth muscle, muscle over which you have no voluntary control but you can feel it cramp now and again, or more regularly if you have something like IBS (irritable bowel syndrome). In my pre-surgery world, occasionally I would feel it move or cramp up the right-hand side of my tummy, which is up the ascending colon, then across the top from right to left, which is the transverse colon, followed by gurgling or cramping down the left side of the tummy, the descending colon, before landing in the rectum and needing the toilet. Now the rumblings and gurglings are all over the place; they are definitely happening, but not in any coordinated way: one loud rumble here, one slightly discomforting huge gurgle there. Not joined up, no obvious synchronization, which makes sense essentially – you touch an organ like the large intestine, cut a bit out and sew it back together and it literally goes and hides in the corner. "Don't touch me! I'm not moving now, just sulking, and now and again I will give a shimmy or a shake." "No, I'm not holding hands with anyone else right now. You moved the person I sit next to. Go away!" I have an uncoordinated, uncontrollable, two-year-old of a gut having a tantrum right now!

Patients don't seem to sleep much in ICU, unless they are sedated. I have another night of slipping in and out of sleep. My family are coming to see me each day: Ben, my siblings, my parents. Ben had packed my favourite childhood book and had promised to read to me each day – as an English teacher he reads aloud really well, with great voices – but even listening to that requires too much concentration. Instead I have the radio on; the radio is like a comforting wave of chat which I don't have to tune into. Or we sit in silence, or rather in the multiple beeps and pinging noises of ICU. I can't do anything more.

SATURDAY 18 MAY

Written in retrospect on Tuesday 21 May

I knew something was wrong. Today I start to get heart-thumping palpitations – it's racing and feels like it's skipping beats. I feel out of myself, out of my body, depersonalized, not in severe pain any longer, but I don't feel right, here in my body.

Getting up the second time is tough, but just as the physio promised, it is far easier than the day before. I was worried I would fail again so the sense of relief when I get up is immense. I celebrated, managing a three-minute walk before going back to bed and a spinning world. The heart palpitations keep happening. Even moving my hand for my phone, or moving my head to look around leads to my heart thumping away in my chest. Not unwell in pain, not unwell in nausea, but in my heart. And now I am so, so afraid. Not of pain, but of my heart stopping. Something else is happening and I am afraid. The doctors explain what I already know, that cutting my organs open, giving me fluids has led to this imbalance of electrolytes that is causing the palpitations and abnormal heart rhythms and rate (tachyarrhythmia – basically a too fast and uncoordinated heart rate). Yet again, my rational head cannot override my emotional one, my doctor head cannot overrule my patient one. We know the cause of this, we can fix this, and yet I am heart-thumpingly afraid, terrified to my very core.

I don't even know what night we are on but it is yet another night of little or no sleep. As the electrolytes go in and the levels of salts in the blood return toward normal the palpitations begin to recede but they are still there. How can you sleep when you feel your heart bumping around in your chest and aren't sure if it is going to keep doing it, when you are terrified that it might forget how to pump entirely and just stop? By 4 a.m. I am so frightened that I don't even know what I want or need any more. And then a doctor does what doctors rarely do. He doesn't immediately try to fix the issue, which is what we as doctors are trained to do: to help, to give a plan to make it better. He simply sits next to my bed, holds my hand and says, "You're having a tough time, aren't you?" He acknowledges me and my situation and then he sits with me. He doesn't give platitudes, doesn't tell me it will be better soon, doesn't even try to make it better now. Instead he sits with me in my fear and discomfort and terror, and that helps more than anything else. In fact, if I learn nothing more from this than the fact that my patients may sometimes need me to sit with them in their pain and fear then I have learned something hugely valuable.

For that short period of time I was not alone, and although the burden of my fear was not lessened, for that moment in time I was not alone in it. He helped me more than he will probably ever know and I don't even know his whole name. And he then gave me medication to make me sleep, for sometimes nothingness is what is needed to allow your mind to rest enough to rest your body. Peace.

Through it all, although incapacitated as a patient, I was still there, so I was still doctoring, or at least trying to think like a doctor myself. I am a GP, I haven't worked in a post-op environment in over a decade, yet it is really hard for me to give up control. The only thing that helps here is chats with the ICU team – we talk in medical language, they tell me what they are doing but inform me as an equal. I need the information in order to be able to give up this control, need the information to know that I am safe.

SUNDAY 19 MAY

Written in retrospect on Tuesday 21 May

I was pretty grumpy yesterday and still am today. In fact, if my family were to read this, they would probably roll around on the floor laughing at how much of an understatement that is. Grumpy, angry and irritable is good; it means that you have enough fight in you, enough energy to feel something, anything at all, even if they are negative emotions. Prior to that I lay listless and lethargic in the bed; even the noise of people talking at normal volume was too loud and the effort of talking myself was enormous.

Today, as the surgeon predicted, I passed wind. But there weren't twenty minutes of excruciating agony prior to it, just the odd huge gurgling, rumbling sensation that I have been having randomly in my tummy which don't seem to be joined up. Even so, I definitely passed wind. How often have you farted and not thought anything at all about it? But for me there was joy, the joy that it didn't hurt, the joy that this means that somewhere, somehow, some part of my bowel has remembered what it is supposed to do and is doing it.

This elation was short-lived as within a few hours I had the delight of soiling myself, which is normal in this situation as your bowel and brain and the sphincter of your anus all have to get reacquainted again. I had no idea it had happened apart from a smell and an odd sensation afterwards. The nurses were kind but it is bad enough lying here not being able to do anything and then having them wipe you over and over and not being in control. "We're used to it," they say, and indeed I know I would say the same to a patient: don't worry, we expect it, it doesn't matter. But it does matter – it matters very much indeed. The nurse is all jolly, saying it is so good as my bowel is working, etc., and all I can think of is that I am thirty-nine and have just pooped myself and a stranger is wiping my bum. I know she isn't judging me, I know I wouldn't judge a patient, and still it is utterly humiliating.

This morning was the first time in my life that I thought that I was actually losing my mind. They were giving me injections of Buscopan to relieve the spasms in my gut and cyclizine for anti-sickness, both of which seemed to bring on the abnormal heart rate, which is a known side effect. I have had cyclizine in the past with no issues but that morning, after they injected me, I had a rather rare reaction. My limbs were jerking uncontrollably, to the point where I would be sitting and suddenly my leg or arm would be thrown about. It led to an enormous and overwhelming sense of panic. I simply could not control myself and was aware of some part of me wondering if this was what it was like to simply lose control, even of your grip on reality. I had no idea whether it was real or a reaction to the psychological stress. Yet most of me just kept panicking, even when the doctor said it was likely to be a drug reaction.

This jerking movement is known as extrapyramidal motor disturbances, which is known to sometimes happen with cyclizine, an anti-sickness medication I was receiving. GPs are not keen on giving medications such as Valium to patients, as they cause addiction and only cover up problems without solving the underlying issue. Yet we do give them, far more rarely in the community than we did even twenty years ago, and they are used, often in psychiatric units or in ICU. There is a time when your mind needs to rest, often in order to allow it and/or your body to heal. And in my case, it needed to physically calm down.

The doses of intravenous diazepam I was given that day allowed me to realize I wasn't going insane. They allowed my heart to slow, which then allowed my panic to fall to anxiety and therefore allowed me to cope. What it also meant though was that I was drowsy when I saw my kids and could only manage five minutes of talking to them. They went off for an ice cream and I only managed a kiss goodbye afterwards. This was the first time I had seen them: the eldest full of conversation of what he had been up to, arms full of thoughtful presents, and though I said thank you I couldn't really express the gratitude and pride I felt; the middlest, smiling shyly but not really engaging; and the youngest silent, just holding my hand. It still makes me sad, that they saw me effectively tied down with my catheter and lines, too tired to be able to lift my head off the bed. I feel sad, and to be honest, a little shame. Which doesn't seem right, but I do; I feel shame that I couldn't be better for them that day.

MONDAY 20 MAY

Today a corner was turned and just for a few minutes I recognized that maybe, just maybe, there would be a tomorrow that wasn't within this room. A room with no natural light, with no day or night, with no sense of time at all, apart from it being long and slow. Time on ICU is interminable: no mealtimes to break it up, no darkness or light, nothing to give you an idea of the passage of time, which is disorientating and infuriating. Time is indeterminate, never, ever ending, and the days and nights merge into one.

Here's the thing about being in hospital: when you are a patient, you wait. In your general everyday adult life, you really don't. Of course you wait for a bus, for dinner to cook, for your partner to phone or whatever, but for tiny everyday mundanities, you do not. Need the loo? Off you trot. Fancy a drink of water? Just stand up and get one. Dry hands? Get up and get some cream. A headache? Have a drink, or a painkiller, or even a rest, but you choose and you simply get on with it.

In hospital and especially in ICU this is not the case. Not because anyone is being mean or trying to torture you, not from malevolence or desire to frustrate, just because they are busy and things take time. I know this. I am not complaining but observing. On ICU if you want to change position and cannot without help you ask; if you want a sip of water, you ask; if you want or need anything, anything at all, things that ordinarily you would not even think about asking for, or even doing, you have to ask. The response is always: in a minute, let me finish the notes I am writing, the medications I am drawing up to inject into your drip, complete the job I am doing and then I will do it for you. On the ward you press your call button and someone comes, sometimes quickly, sometimes less so, but someone comes. Then you make your request, you feel sick, can you have more anti-sickness, and then you wait – for them to get the drug chart, unlock the meds cupboard, get the meds, check the meds with a colleague and then bring them. If you need to leave ICU for a scan, a porter is needed to wheel you down to imaging, where you get parked and left for an indeterminate amount of time to wait, with nothing to do and no one to speak to and after the scan you wait again, parked backward in a waiting room, until someone comes. I do not mean to sound ungrateful, I entirely appreciate that they are doing an amazing job, yet the helplessness is both debilitating and infuriating but mainly just hugely depressing. I am a grown woman – I just want to be able to get myself a drink!

◆

I am getting out of bed far easier than before and shuffling around the ICU unit. What seemed like an impossibility a few days ago is now achievable. Today they put a flip-flop valve on the catheter to train my bladder to remember what it is like to be full again. When the valve is off the bladder fills, and you remember what that sensation feels like, and when you need to go you open it and pee into a bottle rather like those given to old men in hospitals. Who knew I would suddenly be peeing like a man? As a female, I found the whole standing up to urinate idea rather odd, so decided that I'd stick with doing it sitting down on the toilet – after all, my brain is used to weeing when I sit down! I felt like I might need to go and I went. I opened my bowels, soft liquid, stinking and all, but I felt it, I recognized it, I got there and I did it! The same achievement as many two- and three-year-olds up and down this country, but probably the same feelings of relief and joy as felt by their parents!

I sat out for a few hours and then, suddenly exhausted and feeling unwell, I went back to bed. I was sent off for a CT scan to rule out a collection of pus, or an infection from the surgery, as I keep having fevers. So once more I was wheeled around the hospital on a bed, feeling disconcerted by the people who stared at me in lifts and waiting rooms. I saw a consultant I work with there; he gave a double take, checked the name on my notes on my bed and looked away but looked back confused. I called him, saying my professional name, and he hurried over and said that they had discussed my case in the multidisciplinary team meeting last week and he didn't know it was me and how sorry he was and how awful it was. He was kind, he was gentle and the doctor part of me wondered how he or anyone else who knows will ever be able to see me in the same light again. Is this who I am now?

◆

Every day they are giving me a combination of B vitamins and vitamin C through my intravenous lines, called Pabrinex. This is a fluorescent yellow liquid, which also makes my urine look slightly luminescent, and is given to people who aren't receiving these vitamins through food. It is prescribed post-operatively if you are expected not to eat for a period of time, or if you are on haemodialysis for kidney problems, but as a junior doctor I most commonly gave it to alcoholics. If you are getting all your calorie intake from alcohol, or choosing alcohol over food due to your addiction, you aren't getting enough of these vitamins and the deficiency can then cause other problems. As I write this it therefore seems entirely reasonable that I would be having it. I am not getting nutrients from food as I am not eating enough of it so I need them in the Pabrinex. Yet as they hang the bag up each day some part of my brain wonders why I have turned into an alcoholic when I rarely drink at all?

◆

The CT scan shows that there is no infection so I am discharged from ICU to a ward with a window; my brother points out that from my bed I can see the sky. A view of a sky which I haven't seen for what feels like years. I cried. At that moment that sliver of blue represented an outside world, a life, hope. There is an underlying fear and panic which rears its head almost constantly, when alone, in the middle of the night: am I here, am I dying? Will anyone know? In ICU you are constantly monitored – you have one nurse who is there the entire time. On the ward, you think, *Will I be seen? Will you notice if I get sicker?* It is astounding how quickly you become institutionalized.

That night I slept. I slept for about five hours before being awake for about three, in pain, in panic, in worry and alone. I reached for my phone for company, speaking to my brother-in-law, who is away in a different time zone, making connections with other doctor friends abroad. It is the middle of the night and I search for connection – *I am alive, do you know that? Do you feel me? Am I here?* And then mercifully sleep again, natural sleep till the morning.

TUESDAY 21 MAY

Today I have had a shower.

This is not a big deal and yet it is absolutely a momentous occasion. Like all big occasions it is exhausting too! Standing, hooked up with lines in and a catheter, but the simple joy of standing under hot water, washing my hair, my skin, my body (myself!) makes me feel like a human again. I recognize the person in the mirror. Sure, she looks exhausted and drained; yes, her face is strained and her skin looks dry, her lips are peeling and her hair is scraped back. But I am there – somewhere in that rather sick-looking person is me. I am so utterly grateful to see her.

◆

Today we walk, or shuffle up and down the ward, and I struggle to eat. I am now supposed to be on free fluids – everything liquid without bits, juice, consommé, soup, jelly, sweets, milk, yoghurt, ice cream. Only I don't like most of these things. I am not trying to be difficult, but I can't eat consommé; I hate it, it makes me feel nauseous at the best of times and I feel nauseous constantly. The meds, although given intravenously, have a taste and even a flush of normal saline, which is essentially salt water (given before and after medication in an intravenous drip to check that the line is working and to ensure all the medication gets into your body) of the same strength as tears, and make me feel like I have a mouthful of coins. My sense of smell, which has always been good, has been heightened and worsens the nausea. In ICU the smell of the nurses could turn my stomach – not that they smelled bad but just that any scent, even that of another human being, makes me feel sick. Nursing is one of the most intimate parts of care there is – more intimate in a way than the surgery, where the surgeon has their hands inside you while you are asleep. They wash you, they clean you, they see you at your worst and you see them too. I could identify the nurses on ICU by their smells: one smelled of Clarins beauty products, one of eucalyptus-type breath mints, one of their morning coffee.

The dietician has just been and explained that the scan of the previous day showed that there is some jejunal ileus, meaning that part of my small intestine is temporarily paralyzed. This happens commonly after bowel surgery, and explains the nausea. Essentially your bowel should all be moving the contents along but if one part is paralyzed things become blocked and you feel bloated and sick. The second part of my small intestine is still sulking, still on strike from my bowel being handled during the surgery, which results in the nausea. It is temporary, it will pass; currently I struggle on.

So here I am, eating ice cream, frozen yoghurt and milk. My kids, or in fact many people would not understand – after all, I have just had a pot of chocolate ice cream for lunch – what is not to like? The answer is everything! I asked the dietician if I could suck the salt and flavouring off a crisp; she answered only if I promised I wouldn't bite or suck the crisp itself – would you try it or would it be more tortuous to taste the salt and flavour but not crunch the crisp?

After a long period of bowel and bed rest post this kind of surgery, patients will lose weight as they are not eating, and it is important to try to keep up your calorie intake to give your body enough fuel to recover and heal. While on free fluids this is a challenge, so I have to shovel the food in seemingly constantly – milk, frozen yoghurt, disgusting fortified chalky-tasting juice, more milk – but it is just so hard when you feel sick all the time! I long for salt and vinegar crisps, for sushi, even for French toast, which is soft but not quite soft enough.

As the day wore on I trotted, or rather shuffled, up and down the corridor, and even managed a flight of stairs. The thoughts of test results have begun to creep in – when will they come, what will they say? – even though the consultant said it would take about a week, potentially longer. You need to be well enough to worry about what will come next. Up until this point I have just been focused on the now, but the niggle of worry has just begun to creep in.

The next hurdle is for the ureteric stent, the straw which had protected my kidneys, to come out. The urologist appeared and off I went again, being wheeled back down to theatre for the procedure, but on this occasion, by the time I had even worried about having a procedure while I was awake, the catheter was out and a camera was into my bladder. I couldn't help but look on the screen, even though I didn't mean to, remembering last time when I saw the cancer. The stent was obvious, like a straw sticking into the bladder. I heard the urologist say "open" and "close", referring to the surgical tools he was using to grab the stent to remove it. Just as my brain began to register *Oof, it is a bit* – but before I got to finish the thought with *uncomfortable,* it was all over. Yes, there was some spasm and pain afterwards, but for right now that was the last proper procedure, done and dusted. The urologist inserted a new catheter to allow me a night's sleep without worrying whether or not I will pass urine on my own, but it will be taken out tomorrow.

◆

My parents were visiting me that night when the surgeon appeared, said good evening and in the next breath: "All nodes negative. Twenty-seven nodes, all negative." It took me a good few seconds to compute. I had been thinking about it but hadn't expected the results as yet. Negative, he said negative, right? He repeated it, zero out of twenty-seven, all nodes negative. I had to touch him, to put my hand in his in gratitude. I have no idea what I said next, what I did, what was happening around me – all I can remember is the look of relief on my parents' faces. Then the medic-in-me's questions came: the staging, the extent, what next. T3, N0, M0: tumour grade 3, no spread to lymph nodes, no metastases (which means spread of the cancer outside the bowel). All this means that the chances of me needing chemotherapy decrease and all in all gives me a five-year prognosis of survival of 90–95 per cent.

No nodes, no nodes, no nodes.

The lymph nodes are part of your immune system, essentially the traffic lights of your immune system.

Without the spread of your cancer to the nodes, the traffic lights are on red and the cancer can't spread around your body, but once it has spread to the nodes the lights turn green and the cancer can spread to other parts. This is why we remove nodes and why this was about as good news as I could have got at that moment.

The surgeon left and my parents followed so I could call Ben: no nodes, no spread, we got it, it will have gone, even if I need to have chemo, to treat any remnants or seedlings, too small to even be seen at the moment, he got it, he got it all. I could hear the relief and joy down the phone.

It is impossible to put into words what this felt like, to convey the depth of emotion that I felt at that moment. I can say what it means, which is that my chances are really good, that eventually in time this will be a memory and a regular colonoscopy, but to use words to describe how I feel seems impossible. I use words, of course I do, we all use words, but I make part of my living using them, writing them, and I cannot find the words even in my head to express how I feel. This isn't as simple as feeling happy or relieved – these feelings are far bigger than simply one emotion. I just feel all the emotions: sadness, joy, relief, exhaustion. Just feelings, overwhelming feelings. No nodes.

No nodes, no spread. T3, N0, M0.

No nodes!

WEDNESDAY 22 MAY

Doctors lie. We lie all the time, not with malevolent intent, not to harm you, not even by omitting the truth, but by omission of knowledge. Sure, we know that the average length of hospital stay for procedure X is Y, we know the complications and likelihood of having them, we know from patients what hurts and what doesn't, what is uncomfortable and what is actually really sore. Yet we lie, because we don't really know, truly know, what it feels like to be you, to be the patient experiencing the situation and even if we have been through it ourselves we only truly know our experience, not yours. It is why we ask questions of you when we take your history, because you know what we don't, what it feels like, in fact what it is, what is wrong with you; it is generally there in the history, if you know the questions to ask and are able to listen and hear the answers. Take my history: pain, worse two hours before defaecation, which is the pain of the obstruction of the cancer. I was telling you what was wrong even if I didn't know it. Therefore we ask, and you answer and we ask more questions.

I often read patient autobiography type books and recommend them to the doctors I appraise (appraisal is a system that doctors have to go through every year to talk about their continuous professional development, which is how we keep up to date, among other things) as a way of being able to be inside the head of a patient, to learn from their experience. We sympathize, we empathize, but we don't know what it truly feels like, and because we don't know, unknowingly ourselves, we lie.

I knew this was going to be a big operation. I have had surgeries in the past, quite a few of them, and I thought I knew what this would be like. I had no bloody clue and the surgeon just said it was a big operation, major surgery, and I would need one night in ICU. Perhaps I wouldn't allow myself to think what big or major meant; I realize how sick people are when they are in ICU so perhaps I just closed my mind to it. I thought perhaps it would be like the C-sections, which in themselves are no small undertaking but I would be dressed and shuffling off down the ward by the following day. Appendix removal? My partial colectomy laughs in your face! Wisdom teeth removal? My cancer surgery doesn't even deign to compare itself to you.

You see this is a major surgery, but there is no way of conveying what that means. I suppose it is because it is more than muscle, more than cutting through muscle, or even chopping a little bit out, like an appendix, which is vestigial and not even used in our guts.

I recognize the pain of the cuts, the aches in the tummy on walking, the stretching as you lie flattish for someone to examine you, the inability to sleep on your front or even on your side. I recognize these pains, I even welcome them as the knowing is safe: I know I can recover from this.

What I don't recognize is my insides – they rumble, groan and grumble in an uncoordinated way, loudly objecting to the assault on my colon – the nausea and the general sense of being unwell. In touching an organ it temporarily stops working properly and that has an impact on the rest of our carefully coordinated and integrated systems.

I look and feel battered, bruised, like I have been beaten up, but there is a sense that my insides aren't right and I don't know how that improves, I don't recognize this as a healing process – it is new. This recovery is like no other I have experienced, and in living through it perhaps I can begin to understand what my patients have gone through, in that recovery is so much more than your skin and muscles knotting back together.

So I will have lied to patients. "You will get better," I will have said, which isn't a lie. "It will take time," I will have said, again not a lie. But I will also have simply said, "It is a big op and will take time. You are doing well, as well as expected," and I will have tried to reassure them, and in doing so I will have lied, lied from not truly knowing what they were going through.

———————◆———————

I have been allowed to progress to some purée-texture food but low fibre, which is essentially still yoghurt (I hate yoghurt) and thick soups (I hate soup), so for me, milk, ice cream, fortified medicated juices and the like. Mashed up with milk into a purée, I managed half a small variety box size of cornflakes and hours later had horrid pain, nausea and swelling. I cannot be eating enough calories for my needs – it just isn't possible right now. Have a little of what you fancy. Even if I was allowed to, I fancy nothing at all. Is the change that I see in my face weight loss or do I just look haggard, ill and old?

It is amazing how when you just begin to feel better there is space for other niggles to creep in. I keep getting nose bleeds, or even just crusty blood in my nose, probably from irritation from the nasal oxygen prongs which were in for so long (perhaps this is why I spent my junior doctor years putting them back into patients on the geriatrics ward; they always seemed to be resting on their cheeks, not up their noses, oxygenating their cheeks, yet why did we never ask, or they never say?). My gums are bleeding, despite me brushing my teeth many, many times a day to try to get rid of the horrid taste in my mouth from medications, though the constant sucking of sweets, sugar free or not, can't help, or is it just a stress response? I have oral thrush, which actually probably explains the bleeding gums, probably from all the antibiotics, and I have just noticed the irritation that signifies that I have the start of thrush down below too. These are all small irritations, small yet irritating, but that I can notice them is a sign of improvement. Count your blessings and all that? Or just get me a thrush pessary!

───────────────◆───────────────

In the afternoon I escaped. Hospital is one of those places which you can't really leave – you don't go for a little trip out and come back at medicine time! The physiotherapist said I could walk to the park over the road and I was determined, because outside represents everything that is not being inside the hospital. What would you pack for a five-minute walk to a park, a half-hour sit-down in it and a five-minute walk back with your brother as a chaperone? Ordinarily nothing, right? Not the case here. We take water, sugar-free mints for nausea, sugar-filled hard-boiled sweets for an energy boost if needed, a shawl, just stuff. And it was glorious. Yes, I was outside in my pyjamas and a shawl, but to be honest, no one would be banning me from doing the school run or nipping to Tesco in these – no one would know! There is a little park, a haven of green with a kids' playground, a two-hundred-year-old cemetery and some benches around flower beds. A space in which to sit outside, to watch the world go by, watch children and toddlers at play, dogs being walked and humanity just passing slowly through. To remember that there is a world, a non-cancer, non-surgery world, with its own foibles and pleasures was a joy – it was life-affirming.

THURSDAY 23 MAY

I wake up this morning with chest pain, in and under my left breast; it feels sharp and I can't quite catch my breath. The fever, which has never really gone away, has spiked again even higher than expected. Thus we continue the same bumpy recovery pathway that patients all over experience: two steps forward, one back, two steps forward, three back, five forward. As long as the overall trajectory is upward then good and bad days are to be expected, but they are a huge disappointment and today is a worry. The doctors are concerned that there may be a blood clot in my lungs, and an infection elsewhere, so I will be heading back for another scan at some point today.

If I go home tomorrow there is a three-day bank holiday weekend and although I will be given medication to take home I want to be prepared. For example, I have to self-inject a blood thinner for the next month to decrease the risk of developing blood clots so I need a sharps box to dispose of the needles. I am generous as a GP with my cancer patients, in that they often get preferential access, especially at the beginning around diagnosis and initial treatment, and absolutely and particularly when at the end of life. It isn't just cancer patients – it is those who are most needy who get the most time. Yet it is still strange to be on the receiving end with a GP just writing prescriptions without hesitation, for anti-sickness pills, painkillers, my normal medication. She mentioned a sick note, which to be honest as I am self-employed I hadn't thought about, and said she thought she should put down three months. Three months! Three months? I thought I would be back by mid June, early July at the latest. She gently asked what I give patients who have had a one- or two-night ICU stay, and the doctor in me responded, "About two months." "Exactly," she said. "You have had a stay and more." So she put three months with an agreement that we could discuss it again. It felt like a bit of a blow really. I suppose somewhere in my mind, although I know that this recovery is going to be long and slow, there is still a part of me who thinks I will just bounce back when I'm home.

◆

It is 5.15 p.m. and the kids have just left. They came to see me on Sunday in ICU, primarily because we said they would see me that day, but with hindsight I am not sure it was a good idea. Today was so much better and as they came in it was like a light switch was turned on in my world. They all hugged and held me so tightly – quite frankly who cares about pain when it is your kids squeezing and hanging on with all their might? The youngest couldn't let go of me and when I said we could go to the park she asked over and over if I could come too, and over and over and each time when I said I could she replied "Yes!!!" and her smile could light up the moon. The middlest kept coming back for an extra kiss, in between trying out the bed going up and down. As for the eldest, he is the most anxious, the most questioning and concerned: is it safe for me to walk, for me to come home? A never-ending list of questions.

We came back from the park and sat and watched TV for half an hour and the littlest did some colouring – such a normal, mundane half an hour, but for me the most exhilarating and precious thirty minutes I have spent in days. Yesterday I would have said that if something new were found tomorrow that I do not know if I would have the strength to have this operation again. Seeing them today tells me that I would do it tomorrow in a heartbeat, admittedly with a heck of a lot more fear and trepidation, but I would do it without hesitation. I would do anything to be with them. Then the middlest said he hoped I would need chemo as it would be interesting to see bald Mummy! The bluntness of children!

The chest scan was normal, showing no blood clot in the lung, and the pain is most likely muscular from sleeping oddly and shuffling about. This is so much better news than it being a blood clot, which would require more treatment and medication, so bring on the muscular pain – I'll take it! And, since being disconnected from constant drips and antibiotics, the metallic taste in my mouth is receding and the nausea subsiding. In fact, tonight I felt hungry for the first time; of course my eyes are bigger than my ravaged intestines but I managed a small bowel (ha, clearly I have written *bowel* too many times, I mean *bowl*) of low-fibre cereal mashed to purée without either feeling nauseous or having pain later on. It may not seem much, to eat a bowl of cornflakes, but it is this, a series of tiny, almost imperceptible steps which is what makes up recovery.

FRIDAY 24 MAY

Yesterday I finished colouring a picture. Doesn't sound like much, does it? Groundbreaking news: an adult woman does some colouring in! Yet it was the first thing that I have done apart from write this diary since I got here. I have spent much time resting or listening to the radio which acts like a companion, but I haven't had the attention or concentration span, or even the headspace, to pick up a book or watch TV. I only had the energy to lie and listen; the rest of my strength was turned inward, directed at healing.

◆

Yesterday I spent a few hours by myself; I have a husband, two parents and three siblings who have been visiting me, and although lots of other people wanted to see me I was not ready or willing to see them. For the first two or three days the effort of talking was immense and even the noise of other people talking was grating, almost painful, and yet I absolutely did not want to be alone. I was terrified of being on my own, even in ICU, surrounded by nurses. I needed and wanted my family there, not too many of them at a time – even if they were sent to the waiting room while some or other procedure was done – but there, maybe sitting in silence, but there. When I transferred to the ward this fear of being alone took a few days to subside. When they left at night for the first couple of nights I was actively afraid. You become institutionalized. It is normal to become used to being surrounded by on-tap assistance and the change is daunting. Afraid I would die and no one would know, afraid of my feelings, just afraid in general. Yet yesterday felt different and I told them not to rush; it was, as always, lovely to see them, but I didn't need them in the same way. Of course I need them still, and will need lots of help, but the idea of sitting alone for an hour is no longer frightening but appealing.

◆

The dietician came along. She is pleased with my progression to milk and cornflakes. I have been moved to a low-fibre diet, which is the very antithesis of how I eat normally but it feels like huge progress, to manage it without feeling more sick, without extra pain. Being hungry has to be a good sign. This, the improved nausea and the lessening of pain, means that the paralysis of the top of the small intestine must have improved. We knew it would, it just needed time, and that getting up and walking would also have helped.

I am allowed a piece of white toast. White toast is delicious, slathered in butter, hot and crisp from the toaster. I honestly don't know who is more excited, me or the catering manager! She has been so upset that I have not been able to eat; every day she has been asking in a quiet voice, with just a tinge of hope, whether I can have anything new today. She seemed utterly thrilled to make me one slice of white toast. I managed half a piece and it was every bit as divinely delicious as I remember; white toast and butter is veritable manna! Three quarters of an hour later I managed another half – hot, buttered toast is a thing of joy.

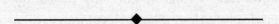

Today I make bail! Not from cancer, from recovery or anything else, but from the hospital, and it is HUGE!!!!! It is not as simple as walking out the door – there are dressings to be changed, the PICC line to be removed, medications to wait for – but by the time the kids get home from school, I will be there. It won't be like nothing has happened, not back to normal, and I'll probably be tired, certainly grumpy, but home, and for them back to being their constant, the base around which their worlds revolve.

I am not sure why being driven home hurts so much; I noticed this before when I had my C-sections. I am walking so my abdomen is used to some jarring every time I put my foot down, yet the bumps in the road are extremely uncomfortable and the journey home seems long. Perhaps you automatically tense your stomach when walking a bit and don't do that flopped in the car?

The irises were out in my front garden when I got home, yellow, blue and purple. They are my favourite flower and although one part of me was saddened that I had missed their burgeoning this year, there is an almost unbearable beauty to them: the richness of the colours, the joyfulness of their splayed petals as they welcome me home. My flowers, my home. I return, tired and sore, perhaps partially broken, but in reality more fixed than before.

Automatically there is an urge to carry on as normal but I know that I cannot, not only physically but not psychologically either. The littlest knows to pat my leg to get my attention instead of my tummy and carefully climbs around me on the sofa to snuggle in front of the TV – bliss.

It is Friday night, time to light my Sabbath candles, which is my time for just a few seconds of contemplation, of prayer, questioning or thanks. Generally I say the blessing, close my eyes, and internally thank God for my children and my family, and ask or beg, *Please, please, keep them happy, healthy and safe*. Tonight I don't even manage that; I close my eyes and the tears stream down my face, and I simply manage "Thank you, thank you, thank you." The family eats and I force down a soft-boiled egg (progress!) and half a piece of toast. I am so, so grateful for their chatter, the tiny rows, hearing about their school day, the mundanities of life.

And so to bed, and the fears start to rise in my head. I am home, I am safe, and yet I am frightened to go to my own bed – not sure of what exactly, just that no one else is there apart from my husband and kids.

Truth be told, once out of ICU and on the ward, I was often the most medically qualified person there. There were nurses and the doctor could of course be called to the ward at any time, but often I would be the most experienced doctor in the ward. I didn't feel responsible for the other patients at all – I most certainly was not in any way, and it would have been a gross breach of confidentiality for me to even know anything about them. In fact, it is only on writing this that it even crosses my mind, but I knew and felt safe that there were other healthcare professionals close at hand and now there are not. My husband has always relied on me to be the doctor, not unreasonably!

I procrastinate, and get slower, taking all my medications carefully (I haven't used that codeine in days and still don't need it now!), giving myself my injection and arranging my nest of pillows. Inside my head I can hear the beep of the call bell, which was a constant backdrop to my hospital days and nights. I settle into bed, grateful to be home, yet anxious at the same time, and fall asleep.

SATURDAY 25 MAY

Last night was the best night's sleep I have had in ten nights. It was not a good night's sleep by general standards but a world away from the constant lights and noise of ICU, or even the disturbance a few times a night on the ward. Hospitals are not great places for sleep, which seems wrong as sleep is essential for healing and recovery. But how can you sleep through the noise and the clatter, the lights on, the blood pressure being taken? Why do they wake you to take your painkillers when you are asleep? Even on the ward I would sleep for a couple of hours and then be awake for two or three long, lonely hours before dropping off for maybe a couple more.

Last night I had about six–seven hours of interrupted sleep. This is a huge amount more than at the hospital, and for some people it may be enough ordinarily, though I am an eight-hour minimum and would really prefer nine. I feel like a superhero in comparison to how I previously did in the morning. A rather slow – no, extremely slow – superhero with absolutely no powers who woke up and then had to lie in bed for an hour to work up the energy to get out of it, but a superhero nonetheless. Sleep, the panacea of health.

Slowly and snail-like, I emerge into the day, showered and in actual clothes for the first time. In getting dressed the differentiation between day and night, between ill health and health, between a mindset of patient and recoveree continues.

The physio was clear: no exercise for at least six weeks, just breathing exercises and gradually increasing walks. Perhaps start at five minutes, he said, and plan the route to think about where there may be a wall to lean on if needed; take it slowly, try to manage three short walks a day instead of one longer walk which then means you can't do anything else the rest of the day. Slow and steady, not boom and bust. In my head this was automatically translated to twenty minutes at least three times daily, which is the doctor in me not listening to being a patient. Surely I as a doctor can do more, surely I with my medical knowledge will be able to do more than an average patient, surely my determination and stubbornness (which is the only reason I manage exercise at all in general) mean that by sheer force of will I can go further and do more than he said? Lots of healthcare professionals feel this when they are patients – feel that somehow they should be super patients, and bounce back quicker than everyone else. This is nonsensical really; knowledge is powerful but it can't make me heal faster.

For the first time, I take steps into the outside world alone, slightly nervously, slowly but savouring the ability to put one foot in front of the other, alone. I compromise with myself at ten minutes, not able to turn off the disappointment of not being the super patient, yet also unable to turn off the need to be the best student and follow directions to the letter (lots of medics are perfectionists – you sort of want us to be, don't you? And competitive too!).

I walk rather like a baby deer, taking its first steps unaided. Not stumbling around, but there is a newness and cautiousness about it, as I gradually stretch my body. Watch a toddler learn to walk and you realize how hard these things are; there is simply so much to think about, keeping upright, standing tall, chest up and head up, and only then keep putting one foot in front of the other. Your instinct is to put your head down and sort of shuffle along, but I follow the instructions, essentially reminding my body how to walk. This leaves little space for thinking, which is probably useful, but there is space to look at the sky, the flowers and plants and revel in their beauty. Simple pleasures, they mean so much.

SUNDAY 26 MAY

Family and friends are wonderful things and I am lucky to have lots of both. There are lots and lots (and lots) of people who care about me, and actually far more than I thought, not necessarily numbers wise but in how much they care.

I kept my phone on silent in the hospital as otherwise the incessant pinging of WhatsApp, texts and messages would have added to the cacophony of noise in there, and also I would have felt a pressure to respond. Instead I stuck to messaging Ben and a group containing my siblings and parents, though that was incessant too, but more of my own doing. This was a real support to me, as if they were really there, all day and night, though they mostly actually were too!

My friends all want to help, everyone wants to help, and now I am home people want to come round. In fact, they wanted to come to the hospital too but bar my closest friend I refused. I wasn't trying to be rude or evasive, just too tired, and while it is acceptable to lie in silence with Ben, my parents or siblings, or even to just hold a hand, it is less so with others!

Perhaps a hundred years ago people would have just come by, maybe even fifty years ago they would have rung first, but now people send a message. There is an element of being removed with a message; they feel they have put the request out into the ether, they feel they have done their bit, but actually that puts the onus on me as the receiver. When can I come, they say? I have no clue. I am literally unable to make that decision. What help do I need? Well, probably some but I don't know what, though I did decide about a morning rota for the kids, but I simply do not have the headspace or capacity to decide what else I/we might need.

Do you want to know how to help your friend with cancer? Don't ask what you can do, don't ask when you can visit, just do something, or come anyway or leave a note. I appreciate that I may sound ungrateful but making decisions and dealing with other people's needs is often almost too much for the person recovering. So decide for us, say, "I am coming on Wednesday at eleven a.m. If that doesn't suit let me know, even if ten minutes before." Don't ask me if I need shopping – I will say no as I don't want to put you out. Instead ring me when you are in the shops and say, "I am standing by the milk and popping by on my way home. Can I get you some?"

Please don't be offended when I don't want to answer all your questions; I can't go over it again and again. Don't push me to discuss what is coming next with treatment as I am not always able to think about it right now. If your friend wants to talk about their illness, then great, your job is to listen, not to offer solutions (unless they ask for them); remember that you used to talk about other things, so do that again.

MONDAY 27 MAY

I have now been injecting myself with Clexane since Friday night. In the hospital they do it for you – every night a small injection into the skin, or fat, generally of the tummy or legs. I need to do this for a month after the operation to prevent blood clots forming in the legs, or worse, pinging off and going to the lungs. Cancer makes your blood sticky. Add to this the almost complete immobility of the first week and relative immobility ever since in comparison to normal, and you are much more likely to get a clot. Which would open up a whole new world of problems that I am not keen to have.

I have no idea how many injections I have given, how many blood tests I have taken, or cannulas I have put in. Not even how many sutures I have thrown, or operations I have assisted in. Lots. But I have never actually given myself an injection. My sharps bin is on my dressing table with strict instructions to the children not to touch or go near it. I have a pile of Clexane injections, which are about as easy to give as an injection can be. There is no need to open vials of medication, to put on one needle to draw it up, then change needles to inject, not forgetting to dispel any air, the steps that I do automatically for someone else. Instead you take off the cover, grab some fat on your belly or thighs, stab the needle in and press the plunger, making sure you don't take your finger off the plunger while you remove the needle, and then chuck the lot in the sharps bin. Easy as pie.

Well, not quite, as everything with me involves questions; even this involves some thought, though in the hospital they literally just grabbed and jabbed. Where is going to be the least painful yet have fat? Not the front of the thigh, surely, as you would be bound to tense, even unconsciously, and therefore be jabbing into muscle, which is not only incorrect but would hurt more. Inner thigh? Surely that would hurt tonnes; another strike off the list. Upper inner arms? Never mind the pain, I'm not sure how you would manage that as you would be one-handed. How can you pinch with one hand and inject with the other if you only have one arm? Bottom? Yes, but again you would essentially be one-handed so that wouldn't work, which only leaves the tummy. My husband said he would do it if I couldn't, or wouldn't, which then opened up the whole landscape of the body again! I braced, then relaxed as bracing would hurt and then allowed the doctor in me to take over. Stop being the irrational patient and allow the calm, detached doctor to take over and get on with the job. The doctor who wouldn't think twice, who would have a running patter going on and be finished even before the patient really noticed. Grab, jab, dispose, done. The thinking is far worse than the doing.

TUESDAY 28 MAY

Having cancer is like getting continually, repeatedly punched in the face. "The biopsies confirmed colon cancer", KAPOW, punch to the face, fall down, get up. "You need major surgery", SPLAT, blow to the kidneys, fall down, get up; "You might need a bag", KAZAM, right hook to the stomach, fall down, get up; the nodes, the pain, BANG, POP, SPLAT, KAPOW, fall down, fall down, fall down, get up, get up! Get up, keep going, head down, listen, ask questions, keep going, have your tests, have your surgery, get strong, keep going, keep moving. No other option, keep walking, one foot then the other, over and over again until the day is done.

Today I am seeing the oncologist, though I have been thinking about it for days, thinking about chemotherapy. I have no spread, no nodes and he got all the cancer out, so R0 (resection zero). We use chemotherapy to treat cancer, but also to prevent cancer coming back, to treat tiny seedlings too small to be seen and removed surgically and kill them off, to stop them being able to blossom into a recurrence of cancer. Some part of me isn't sure why I am going. The surgeon said I should, but that he thought the chances of chemo were now small, that he got it all.

◆

That was a blow… or rather a few blows. In my head I thought they would say no chemo needed, and that I would struggle somehow with that, even the idea of my cancer being truly done, as this whole period is so huge and unprocessed for me right now, but he didn't say that at all.

I knew that for where I am, my exact cancer – T3a, N0, M0 – the five-year survival rate is 90–95 per cent. I knew that. What I had not thought about at all was the recurrence rate, the chances of the cancer coming back. Stupid of me really, but I just haven't had the headspace to think clearly. After all, the five-year survival rate depends on lots of things, mainly whether or not the cancer recurs! If it recurs, it doesn't mean that you won't survive, but that more treatment, etc. is needed. The oncologist talked about recurrence and while I hadn't considered it at all, from the moment it came out of his mouth to the ten seconds later when he told me what the figure was, it never occurred to me that the number would be as high as he said.

T3a, N0, M0, R0 (the numbers and letters I keep hanging on to as they are really quite good, though maybe just not good enough) has a 20–30 per cent chance of recurrence. He said taking into account everything about the operation, the histology (what the cells looked like when examined under the microscope), my age, general health, etc. that I was probably at the lower end of this, the 20 per cent end.

Perhaps to you that sounds good, in the same way that a 10–17 per cent chance of needing a bag meant that I was more likely to not need one. But I remember just before I went for my colonoscopy the surgeon said that there was a 1 per cent chance of him finding a polyp in someone my age, and of that a 1 per cent chance it would be something he couldn't remove, like a polyp. That is 1 per cent of 1 per cent, as in 1 in 10,000, so you will forgive me if 20 per cent seems astonishingly high. I appreciate probability doesn't work like that, that for each roll of the dice the odds are the same, but while I understand that intellectually, emotionally it doesn't make sense. If I was the 1 per cent of the 1 per cent, why wouldn't I also be in the unlucky 20 per cent with recurrence?

With chemotherapy, the chances of recurrence are reduced by… wait for it… a whopping 3.5 per cent. 3.5 per cent. Assuming I have a 20 per cent chance of recurrence, with chemotherapy that is reduced to 16.5 per cent.

I had no clue. As both a patient and doctor, I assumed the number would be far higher, that if I had chemo it would be reduced to something really low like 2 per cent or even 5 per cent, that if it were offered to me that the decision would be a no-brainer. The oncologist continued to say that a 3.5 per cent reduction with chemotherapy is considered a good result. Who knew? I didn't and I am a frigging doctor. Admittedly I'm not an oncologist, which is why we are here, but I did not know that the numbers were so small.

Still, you can't decide yet, on the numbers alone. You can't balance the pros and cons on your medical scales, weigh up the potential risks and side effects against potential gains until you know what the risks and side effects are.

◆

The oncologist advised single agent chemotherapy. The agent is 5FU (fluorouracil), which can be given intravenously or orally in tablet form (called capecitabine) for six months. If you take it orally, you take it twice daily for two weeks then have a week off and repeat for the six months. If you choose intravenous, then you have a long-term line called a port inserted into your chest, and would come in every two weeks to be hooked up to an infusion which you would then go home with for forty-eight hours before returning to have it removed and see the doctor fortnightly.

Practicalities of how to even take the drugs aside, we move on to side effects. 5FU is a pretty old drug so we know about the side effects quite well and although the oncologist went through them he also gave me leaflets to read later. He said that it is generally pretty well tolerated and some people have no side effects at all but others struggle. The list of potential side effects include:

- Dropping your white blood cell count and therefore being at risk of infection.
- Fatigue – he said this was the biggie here.
- Nausea and/or vomiting – but this should be controlled with other medication.
- Sore, red palms of your hands and soles of your feet.
- Sore mouth.
- Hair thinning – but hair falling out entirely was rare.

I asked about hair loss and apologized for my own question, saying that I knew it shouldn't matter but that it did. He batted it straight back, saying that of course it matters to me and whatever matters to me matters to him. It may well thin, but not all come out. As I write this I think, *What does that mean?* As much as after my babies, which really was quite a lot, or more? In patches or generally? And it won't just be the hair on my head but my eyebrows too. Should I do microblading? (I mentioned this to Ben afterwards, and he seemed more distressed by the idea of a semi-permanent tattoo of my eyebrows being too heavy than the idea that they might be patchy!)

Importantly, he states that the oral tablets are more likely to have side effects than the infusions, but, if they are well tolerated, fit in easier with everyday life, and if the side effects of the tablets are too great then we can change to the intravenous version. Despite having fewer side effects, the intravenous version is more time-consuming and therefore burdensome. He also mentioned that he would give the same response if I were twenty years older, so the decision about chemotherapy was not simply based on my age.

I know that ultimately this decision is mine, that no one is going to tie me down and forcibly inject me with chemotherapy, but I desperately want to be guided, I want a little paternalism, I want to feel safe and looked after. I want someone, if not to tell me what to do, then to help me decide. So I told him that. He has a very considered, thoughtful manner and his exact words were: "On the balance of all things I would recommend it". He had me at the words "on the balance" – as a doctor everything is a risks vs benefits balance, a weighing up of the evidence. He is a man who speaks my language.

If there is a chance, any chance of there being something to reduce the risks of this cancer coming back, then I have to take it. Apparently the greatest risk of recurrence is in the first two years but I would never forgive myself, on behalf of my children, if I didn't do something which could help and the cancer then came back. So actually there is no choice, and although it is a disappointing blow, and awful, and unfair, I still have to do it.

The outcome of this consultation was for me to go home, get strong, get pain-free and recover and reassess in two weeks, but essentially my decision is made.

As for my cancer, it isn't quite done yet. I thought he would have been incinerated by now, but apparently not. For a while he is kept, not alive as such – he was never sentient, which somehow makes it worse, that I was growing this thing which wanted to take over and kill me, but without any reason at all. He is probably frozen somewhere. But if most of him has been incinerated, bits of him on slides are frozen and kept in a hospital lab somewhere and will be taken out and examined further to help us decide exactly which chemo is required, and if it is more likely that I have a particular syndrome or not. In my mind I prefer to imagine that he is whole with tiny bits being slivered off him as he protests wildly, trying not to give up his devious information, but he is kept, bound and gagged, to be for our use now – all his information is now to help me, not harm.

Interesting. I appear to have given the cancer a gender now. Actually I just wrote "my cancer" and went back and changed it to "the cancer"; I don't want it to be mine! Why in my head is the cancer a "he"? This isn't a comment on men – it is just another way of separating it from my identity, from myself. If I am female then it can be male. It is from me but not me – it helps me keep them separate.

WEDNESDAY 29 MAY

A tale of two bowels (or a tale of two shitties – at least I amuse myself!):

Up until two weeks ago I thought I knew my body. I knew when I was hungry. I knew when I felt a bit sick when it was hunger, when it was nerves or fatigue, when it meant I was unwell or when it was pregnancy. I knew when I needed to go to the toilet to do a poo, when I could hold on for the next patient, or next three patients or even the whole morning (don't do that – it actually makes you more constipated). I may have been constipated, like many people are, especially women, but I knew my normal. If I ate lots of fibre, fruit and veg, golden linseeds (excellent for constipation – take two tablespoons a day, sprinkle it on your cereal or yoghurt), exercised and drank lots of water I would go most days. And when things got a bit worse, for example, when I went on holiday, I would take a laxative to help things along. It may not have been perfect but my bowel was mine and we had an understanding of each other.

At least I thought I did, though perhaps not, as it was growing a malevolent being inside me. I didn't have the classic symptoms of bowel cancer, such as a change in bowel habit, but even if I had become slightly less constipated I would simply have thought that my diet and lifestyle were working, that the linseeds were doing their job! Unless I suddenly developed diarrhoea all the time, I simply wouldn't have thought about it. We think of a change in bowel habit as getting diarrhoea where there wasn't any before, or vice versa, but not hugely constipated compared to a little less constipated – even if this did happen, all you would feel would be relief!

So that was me, my guts and my poop, muddling along with each other before.

That was my bowel pre-op. This is now.

We don't know each other at all.

I have no recognition of my body and I am not talking about what it looks like. I mean what it does, how it works and when it wants to go. I didn't feel hungry for at least seven days after the operation, and had absolutely no desire to eat at all, despite having to constantly eat ice cream and drink milk. Feeling hungry was a new experience – before that I just felt sick all the time – but I noticed that toward the end of that first week there were periods when I felt weaker than others, which may have meant that I needed to eat something.

I now feel hungry but often when I eat I feel nauseous and bloated and can only eat small amounts at a time. I used to be a bit of a grazer as I never could eat big volumes but I knew when I was hungry, and mostly knew why I was eating, because I was bored, or cross, or sad, or tired. I don't know any of that now.

As for my bowels, we are like strangers at the moment. In the first few days after the surgery, when I was waiting for the all-important first fart, I would wish and hope and pray that the two parts of my bowel would join together and that the join would remain intact. Then once we were past that point, it brought me to the most humiliating moments I have experienced: not being able to control liquid vs air and having to clean myself up, or rather be cleaned up after an accident.

I then thought we were coming to some sort of an understanding as by the next day I knew I needed to go to the toilet and was so proud of my guts when I was able to pass a small amount of liquid stool each time. A combination of the surgery, constant antibiotics and one ICU doctor prescribing laxatives (to the horror of the surgeon) meant the following two or so days resulted in diarrhoea at least twelve times a day, but the last few days in hospital it was only twice, which is manageable.

And then my bowels stopped – stopped entirely. It is now Thursday and I have not done more than a pellet since last Friday night. My bowel is on strike again, back hiding in the corner, refusing to come out of its bedroom to join in and play. There is always a concern about developing bowel obstruction, where there is a complete blockage of the bowel after surgery due to scar tissue, and it means you can't pass wind and tend to vomit. I have been passing gas and haven't vomited, therefore I know that I am not obstructed. This is not an emergency, but I can't poop! I know I need to go, but I can't. And it hurts, it really hurts.

I am taking a laxative and know it takes about six weeks for the bowels to settle down and to work out what your new normal is. I thought that if some of my colon was removed I would never be constipated again; currently this is wrong!

THURSDAY 30 MAY

I am being looked after by both a surgeon and a physician; both are doctors but they are very different breeds of doctor. We divide ourselves into our relative surgery or medicine tribes quite early on; people tend not to know which way they want to go as medical students but have generally decided by the end of their first jobs as the most junior doctor. At that point you choose your specialty training – medicine, surgery, paediatrics, obstetrics and gynaecology, psychiatry, general practice or others – and within those are the two tribes, surgeons and medics.

General surgeons may later specialize into vascular surgeons, or orthopaedic or other, or be gynaecologists, but anyone who operates is a surgeon. Everyone else is a medic and traditionally does not operate at all; instead they deal with medicines. We are very different beasts, in what we do, how we do it, the risks we take and when we take them – essentially in who we are. Medics heal with medicine: take this medicine – it may help, it may not, we know that if X number of people take this, Y number will improve, while Z number may not so let's try; or take this medicine to help you stop getting something else in the future. It is a lot less immediate, with fewer immediate outcomes or satisfaction that you can see in such an obvious way.

General practice again is slightly different: sure, I can do the odd procedure here or there, insert a coil, remove lumps and bumps or do joint injections, but we generally use medicines and most importantly we use time, and often ourselves, to simply offer support while the body and mind heal. I have many a patient who comes to check in with me; I am not sure that I do much else but reassure them, yet interestingly that seems to be enough for them, and for me.

Surgeons heal by cutting, by fixing, taking out the bad bit and either letting the body heal or replacing the defective part: broken hip, we'll give you a new one; worn-out knee, here's a nice replacement; appendix giving you gyp, I'll just get rid of that then. Cancer? I'll just whip that out.

Surgeons are sometimes called arrogant, used in a negative way, and it is said that they can have a God complex. Of course they are arrogant – that arrogance is essential for their jobs. It takes a certain level of confidence to hold a scalpel in your hand and know in the very core of your being, in the soul of who you are, that you can cut the person prostrate on the table in front of you in order to heal them. That you are going to hurt them, really cause them pain, and that there are risks involved in the procedure ahead, yet knowing that it is for the best, that you can help them, you can cure them.

It is a fallacy that all doctors take the Hippocratic oath, a traditional doctor's oath swearing to uphold certain ethical values. I certainly didn't and know very few colleagues who did on graduating medical school; some took a more modern version, most took nothing, though we all have to subscribe to the duties of a doctor set out by the General Medical Council, the body that oversees doctors.

Firstly, the classic version requires you to swear by Apollo the physician, Asclepius, Hygieia, Panaceia and, as far as I am aware, the Ancient Greek gods have somewhat fallen out of fashion. There are some values and premises that are definitely still relevant today – the need to respect the teachers who taught you the art of medicine, and to promise to pass this on – but it also states you can't perform an abortion.

Perhaps the most famous concept attributed to the Hippocratic oath, *"primum non nocere"*, "first, do no harm", is not even in there but is from another work written by the Greek physician Hippocrates, called *Of the Epidemics*. "First, do no harm" cannot apply to medicine if taken in absolute terms. We do harm all the time; I hurt you when I take a blood test, and even if I don't put the needle in myself, I know that by filling in the form you are going to get hurt. I know that you may experience side effects from the drugs I prescribe, but if we feel the benefits outweigh the risks you get prescribed them. And when we operate we harm, to do good for sure, but you cannot subscribe to "first, do no harm" if first harm is for a second good.

It takes a certain arrogance to hold a scalpel, to cause bleeding, to hold blood vessels in your hand and clamp them to turn off the blood supply while you work, to remove a cancer, remove the rotten bit of piping and sew the lot back together and expect it to work again. You need that confidence to start, to cut into a living body, to believe you will do good. Surgeons should not have a God complex – they aren't the divine – but to walk away at the end of the day and know that you removed my cancer, that you saved my life? That is worthy of pride.

Yesterday I saw my surgeon for my post-operative review and the removal of staples from my wounds. I asked how I would have presented if this wasn't detected when it was; would it have been in a few years with metastases, or earlier? He felt I would have gone into obstruction, a surgical emergency where the bowel is completely obstructed and nothing, not even air, can pass through. I was partially obstructed before the diagnosis. The outcomes from emergency surgery are never as good as for elective surgery – the likelihood was that I would have needed a far bigger surgery (and this was already pretty huge), with a bag which may not have been temporary. I am grateful I presented when I did, though now, with hindsight, I wish I had presented earlier.

And then he admitted his fears, his worries about the surgery, how he considered a bag but took a risk and then worried for days as I continued to spike fevers in ICU. That he worried about my heart rhythm, that he just worried. Now, thankfully for me, he has moved on to worrying about someone else!

There is a need to somehow convey my gratitude toward him. How do we as patients tell our doctors how thankful we are? I know I like receiving thank-you cards, often from those you least expect, or from those you don't even remember going the extra mile for! Just saying thank you though doesn't seem enough – he has saved my life. I put my hand out to shake his, in that rather English, understated way. He opened his arms and we hugged, simply, thank you.

I will never forget my surgeon. I will never not be grateful to him.

FRIDAY 31 MAY

Last night before bed I made a mistake. I looked at Ben's phone, browsing the pictures from when he took the children to a funfair this week. But I got sidetracked by the photos of the wounds, which I asked him to take as I wanted to see them properly, and photos from the hospital. I had no idea how half dead I looked, slumped while propped up in an ICU bed, tied to the bed by wires and lines. I remember the first photo he took, on the first evening post-op and remember giving him a thumbs up. I think I thought I was OK, doing all right; I look horrendous in that photo. In the photos that follow my brow is furrowed against pain, or my lips are set together as I prepare to stand while being assisted by two nurses. I look drawn, I look like I hurt, I look terrible.

My upset wasn't about what I looked like as such, not the dark circles under my eyes, that I was wearing a hospital gown or that my hair was scraped back, but about the expression on my face, of pain, of determination, the effort to do the simplest of things (which even now are so, so much easier), and just how generally unwell I looked.

My sadness was not even for me, but for him, and for my parents, siblings and children. I went upstairs to him and apologized. He said I shouldn't apologize, that I had nothing to be sorry about. I must have put them all through hell – I still am probably putting them through pain and sorrow – I just didn't realize how bad I looked and how awful it must have been for them to see it. They came in with concerned looks or big smiles and told me I was OK; I think they lied!

◆

Today is the end of half-term and the kids are all back to school on Monday. I think that this will actually be far easier for all concerned. I love my kids, of course I do, but even the noise level going up is tiring, and although everyone is being gentle, there are the constant demands of being a mother.

I am ashamed to admit it, but definitely for the first night after the op and the first day there were hours I did not think of my children at all. On the day of the operation, once I had spoken to them in the morning, I very firmly put them out of my head when I went down to the pre-op room. You aren't allowed pictures in ICU, so their drawings did not even go up on my bedside table till I was on the ward.

Why am I ashamed? Surely hours pass in normal life where I don't think of them? This felt different. When a photo beeped on my phone, or when I was back on the ward and it suddenly occurred to me it was 5 p.m. and I should phone them, I felt guilty, guilty for them not being in the forefront of my mind.

If I admit this to anybody they will say that I knew they were safe, knew they were whole and well, and that I had to focus on myself. Rationally I understand that, but it felt very different to normal life and for hours in hospital they simply did not cross my mind. Nor did anything really. I didn't watch TV, didn't read a book, and my family often sat with me in silence. I can't even say that my focus was internal, on getting well; it felt like I had no focus at all. There was no thought about getting better, no concentrating on being well, no visualizations, just mindlessly going forward, putting one shuffling foot in front of the other, over and over again. This acceptance and determination *was* me getting better, yet I feel guilt about my children.

Now I am home and although I am present, I am a present parent as opposed to an active one. I am here for cuddles – though climb around me and hug me gently – mealtimes and stories before bed, but for much of the time, although I am present in the house, I am not very engaged or remotely as active a parent as I usually am.

It takes me so long to get dressed, then I have to walk and though one or more of them may accompany me, there is a definite awareness that the walk is for me and not a fun scoot or walk to the park for them. I need a rest and sit on the daybed writing this diary, while they play in the garden, or the littlest colours at my feet, the eldest tries to do quiet activities that maybe I could also do, and the middlest asks for a game of cards. We sit, we play, and soon I will get back to being the parent I want to be, just not as quickly as I want it to be.

Ben is being the active parent, doing the household chores, managing the everyday arguments, hurts and nags, preparing meals and doing bath time, and I sweep in at bedtime to do some reading. He is the active parent and I am present, which I suppose is better than being the absent parent, but I am not sure it is good enough. This isn't to put Ben down – I am not a better parent than him, we parent together, we manage the house together – but right now he is doing more than normal. It is probably good for them to have a change, but for me, being a present parent adds to the guilt that I feel around having cancer.

It is bad enough that I am putting my children through this experience. It is awful that because of me and the cancer I have they will have to have regular colonoscopies from early adulthood, even though this will protect them. I feel guilt that they have been upset by this, I feel shame that I put them through this, yet none of this was done consciously or on purpose; I feel guilt but it isn't my fault.

I subscribe to only one theory of parenting, called the "good enough" theory by the paediatrician and psychoanalyst Donald Winnicott. This theory says that you don't have to be a perfect parent, that if you are too perfect your child will never come to understand the frustrations of life, will never become independent as they have no need to become so. I have then further interpreted this in my head to mean that if you do your best and love your children, you will be good enough for them – perhaps not for someone else's children, but for yours. Right now, I do not feel that I am being good enough.

SATURDAY 1 JUNE

My pain deteriorated yesterday, and pressing on the largest incision made it worse. I could not lie on my left-hand side despite before then being able to prop myself up a bit sideways. I was still passing urine, gas and a small amount of rabbit-like stool, but I felt ill, had a fever and the pain wasn't controlled with my normal painkillers. It is impossible to stop your mind wandering off down worst-case scenario avenue: is the anastomosis (the join) breaking down, is there a collection or abscess there, is there a leak, will I need that bag?

The combination of pain, constipation and anxiety led me to a dark head place. I proceeded to eat my feelings and consumed a bag of chocolate raisins (despite being told to avoid dried fruit still) and a bag of chewy sweets. This of course didn't help but no point beating myself up about every tiny thing right now. I started fixating on hair thinning, on fatigue, on every little side effect of the upcoming chemotherapy and was only comfortable if I lay entirely still. I could see I was frightening Ben, that he was unhappy that I was unhappy, but I couldn't stop it.

I went to bed and slept for three hours before being woken by the pain. On changing my dressings I realized that the skin around the largest incision is red, hot, swollen and tender, the four classic signs of infection. I have a slight fever and my pulse is a bit fast, but now I know what is going on, and that it is treatable, my anxiety instantly recedes into the background. Once I am more in control I can see that Ben's anxiety does too, though it is still there. He needs me to be in charge on the medicine front; as long as I know what is going on and can make decisions about it he is fine. I suppose he prefers it when I am doctor, not patient! After seeing the doctor, I was started on antibiotics for a wound infection.

One expects or hopes recovery to be a linear incline back to health, no matter how shallow the gradient of that incline. It isn't. There are ups and downs, and bumps in the road – frustrating, angst-inducing bumps – and it is this constant roller coastering which is so, so difficult emotionally, for Ben as well as me. I have a need to keep progressing forward, and at an ever-increasing rate; stalling even momentarily, or going backward slightly, feels like falling into a ravine, or sometimes a ravine with water in the bottom, or one with spikes or bears in. It all feels catastrophic. Sometimes the climb back up will be as quick as the fall down; other times it will be slower.

It is definitely easier doing this recovery and recuperation when the weather is nice! I spent the afternoon in the garden, with my feet in the paddling pool, with the children. After an hour or so they had moved on to other things and I spent the rest of the afternoon lying on the swing seat watching the breeze ruffle the leaves on the trees. Rather like when you put a baby on a mat under a tree in the summer and they seem fascinated, watching the light and the leaves. Not reading, not on my phone, just being, listening, breathing. This was not a conscious decision to be mindful, to meditate or relax, but a combination of fatigue, being unwell and not being able to do more. But for this afternoon, just being was enough.

SUNDAY 2 JUNE

If previously we had a tale of two bowels, we now have a tale of about four diets.

First there was my normal diet, and by the word *diet* I mean what I put in my mouth each day as opposed to a restrictive diet as such. I know I am fortunate to have a body type which society deems acceptable, although I do have to work at it and generally stick to the 80:20 rule: 80 per cent of the time I try to eat a healthy, balanced diet and that means that 20 per cent of the time it doesn't matter if I eat whatever I want.

The second diet of my four was bowel prep and then bowel rest, gradually increasing my intake of water. The third was progressing to free fluids and then clear fluids, meaning yoghurts, milk and ice cream. You would have thought I would have liked it – what's not to like about ice cream? But the constant sweetness plus the metallic taste and nausea meant it was incredibly hard.

When I was discharged from hospital, I was put on a low-fibre diet, or diet number four. I was given a sheet of allowed foods and told to introduce them gradually and to eat small amounts regularly. This diet is the antithesis of how I normally try to eat. All the white carbs are allowed – bread, pastry, biscuits, pasta, rice, etc. – as well as all dairy, fish, meat and poultry. I'm also allowed cooked and stewed apple, pear or peach, raw peeled apple, tinned fruit bar pineapple, cooked root veg, lettuce and peeled cucumber. Most vegetables – or, importantly, how I enjoy my vegetables, which is mainly raw – are not allowed, with no berries and extremely little fruit in general. No peas, no corn, no, no, no. No nuts, no seeds, no dried fruit, nothing that I would ordinarily snack on, no, no, no. No whole grains, only sugary cereals, not high-fibre ones, not even 50:50 loaf.

I have to eat small amounts regularly and shouldn't add more than one new thing in a day, so I know what is agreeing with me and what isn't; if you eat too much fibre there will be pain and bloating. Essentially, I was told to go home and start trying to gradually increase both the volume and variety of what I'm eating.

Generally I think I spend quite a lot of time thinking about what to cook, who likes what, what I can make out of the contents of the fridge, but this was another level, constantly thinking about food, what to eat, what I could eat and how to keep up my calorie intake.

It is like reverse weaning a baby somehow, though you don't generally give a baby chocolate ice cream for a week! There I was, weaning myself away from mostly milk to cornflakes, then white fish and peeled cucumber and avocado for lunch. I was allowed white carbs but wanted to get protein and vegetables in before I became too full to eat more. As the days have gone by, I have been gradually introducing chicken, rice, other fish and very, very gradually have introduced cooked veg and stewed apple. My sluggish bowel needs to heal but it also needs fibre in order to poo, so I continue with lots of laxatives.

There are many reasons why we tell patients, or indeed everyone, to eat lots of fruit and vegetables, to have a high-fibre diet with whole grains. Aside from the myriad of health benefits that fibre has, including reducing your risk of bowel cancer (oh, the irony!), fibre keeps you full.

In the first few days at home I would have cornflakes for breakfast, a glass of milk and rich tea biscuits at about 11 a.m., white fish and avocado for lunch, then ice cream and/or toast or crumpets at teatime, before eggs and a piece of toast for dinner, with maybe a quarter of a peeled apple.

The further along the line I go, the more I recover, the hungrier I become. I am now at the point of cereal or white toast for breakfast, fish or chicken with some roasted mixed veg (squash/carrot/parsnip/courgette) for lunch and then a small portion of whatever is being had for dinner with adjustments, maybe a meatball with some white rice, or a small amount of Bolognese and white pasta.

I am trying to gradually get back to diet number one, my original lifestyle, and to increase the vegetables, but on the one day I have had veggies at lunch and dinner as well I regretted it, with bloating and abdominal pain. I manage a piece of fruit and am gradually trying to add in a bit more, or a piece with the skin on. I even think I may be going too quickly, which may be contributing to the bloating and pain, and tomorrow will cut those vegetables in half. And in between, when I am hungry, I eat whatever white carb or junk food there is; chocolate is allowed!

It feels wrong. I have just had a major surgery, I am about to go into chemotherapy, and I feel I should be eating as healthily as possible: lots of fruit and vegetables, lots of whole grains and protein and healthy fats. I had so many antibiotics in hospital, and was given an oral course yesterday for the infection, that my gut microbiome (the bacteria present in the gut) will be depleted. I lost muscle mass and in order to regain this, and to heal properly, I need to eat protein. This is what I feel I should be eating. What I have been consuming isn't what I am used to, or what I think suits my body best – it feels strange!

I am impatient, impatient to start eating again in the way I enjoy, in the way I feel nourishes my body. There is no joy in eating biscuits right now – somehow the pleasure has been taken away. All these things – what you like to eat, when you eat, how you eat – are part of who you are, and all of these things have changed.

MONDAY 3 JUNE

There is a simple joy and satisfaction in doing a poo; we should all appreciate such things. Needing to go, going without a huge amount of pain and then feeling empty, this simple pleasure should be noted. I have begun to go, albeit in small amounts, with discomfort (actually I lie, initially with hang on to the sink and pant pain), and while I don't feel empty I know that progress is being made. Albeit with a load of laxatives, but I am getting there! At some point I may well go completely the other way, but right now there is just a huge relief in going at all!

Last night I lay in Ben's arms and the tears began to flow. Yes, I have cried since this diagnosis, cried all the bloody time really. Cried in shock, cried in fear, cried in panic and anxiety, cried in pain, cried for my kids, cried in shame, cried imagining what would come next. Last night I cried with real sadness, sadness for everything that has been and is still to come. I cried with frustration, I want to be better now, I want my body to feel like itself again, I want to not hurt, I want to be well quicker. And finally I cried because it just isn't fair, for my husband, my kids, my family and for me.

I am a pragmatic person, a realist. While I appreciate the impact that your brain can have on your body I also think that sometimes you need to feel the lows, in order to experience the highs. When people tell you to only think positively, to not focus on the past or the bad days sometimes, and often unwittingly, they belittle your experience. Sometimes you need to shout and rail against the unfairness of it all, against the world. Last night what I needed, and I didn't even know I needed it until I was soaking Ben's shoulder with my tears, was to allow myself to feel whatever it was I was feeling, which last night was both frustration and sadness. Sometimes you just need to marinade in the sheer awfulness of your situation in order to be able to pick yourself up again and carry on. At least that is true for me.

TUESDAY 4 JUNE

Today I went to my first physio session. This is to try to prevent adhesions (internal scar tissue sticking your organs together) forming again from the surgeries as well as extraordinarily slowly beginning to get me to stretch and move. It may also help the appearance of the scars, one of which is extremely lumpy and hard, but that isn't its primary aim. Essentially it involved painful abdominal massage – as they massage they cause tiny little traumas to the scar tissue to break it up. It takes time but can mean that you end up moving easier, without pain. Having someone massage your tummy is a slightly strange experience – it isn't somewhere which would normally be rubbed in a massage and this isn't a gentle relaxing massage but a grinding, kneading, painful one!

Scar tissue can remodel for up to about a year, so you won't know what your scars will look like on the outside, or feel like on the inside, for a really long time after surgery. This doesn't mean that I will need physio for that long – just until my mobility is back to normal and I don't have pain on movement. When a surgeon cuts your abdomen they cut into your core muscles, the ones whose job it is to hold you up, and you have to rebuild that strength, slowly, slowly over time. I want my body to be healthy – no, I *need* it to be healthy – in all the ways it can be. Yes, the surgery will change me, I will carry scars, but this physio will help me heal, so painful or not, I continue.

I now feel slightly sick. See you next week!!

WEDNESDAY 5 JUNE

As a society we have lost the art of convalescence. Convalescence is the time spent recovering or recuperating after an illness, which is essentially what I am doing, or am supposed to be doing, right now. In fact, I did a piece with Vanessa Feltz on her BBC Radio London breakfast show about convalescence recently so have really thought about this. Fifty or a hundred years ago medicine was not as advanced as it is now, and without antibiotics or with less sophisticated surgery often the only answer was to rest and let the body heal. There were convalescent homes up and down the country, often on the coast for the sea air, and people would go and spend weeks or even months at a time in one, recovering after a bout of flu or an operation. A stomach ulcer, which is now treated with medication, was treated with a diet of milk and rest, as were many other illnesses. Medicine has moved on. Low back pain is no longer treated with bed rest but with movement; in fact, getting up and about is important for all illness and recovery, as sitting or lying too long increases your risk of deep-vein thrombosis. Not everything about convalescence would now be considered correct, but the concept of it is still relevant.

Now we expect far more from medicine: we expect there to be an answer for everything, a magic pill to make everything OK, whether or not they actually exist. And while we have medications for various conditions and can perform complex, intricate, life-saving surgeries, we still seem to expect life to get back to normal straight away, and it does not.

In our 24/7 society, where everyone is switched on all the time (which we know is not good for you), everyone thinks that once their operation is done their bodies should simply ping back, both in function and looks. Even if you do take time off work, it is exceptionally difficult to truly turn off, not to answer emails, or be involved in a conference call. Some of this pressure may come from work, which it should not if you are on sick leave, but much of it comes from ourselves. We feel if we don't respond or stay involved that we will be forgotten somehow, or that we will be considered less — less of a team player, less of a hard worker, just less. Whatever it is that we do that contributes to who we are as a human, as a person, seems to be immensely important and I know I worry that to do less of those things somehow diminishes me.

Therefore there is a constant struggle: the need to be a good mother vs the fact that I get grumpy and irritable the more tired I am; the need to be involved in the mothering even though it is exhausting; in order to be able to parent I have to accept that I can't do the laundry or other chores. The need to still be a doctor, which is a really significant part of my identity, vs the need to rest and the fact that, even if you ignore my body, my brain simply will not move as quickly as it used to while I heal and that I am not sure that right now I would be clinically safe to work (so I am not!).

I compromise by writing my magazine copy, and planning when I will go back, and even by writing this diary. Writing a section each day feels like I have achieved something, and no matter how small, it is something. I want to still do charity work but have no time, energy or headspace to give; I had to give up the school governing-body work, but I won't give up the Jo's Cervical Cancer Trust work, I can't give up more. I have a desire to work out and feel healthy and good about myself, which battles the fact that my body simply would not do it, and more than that I would be likely to cause harm by striding back into a HIIT session. Actually, the decision about whether or not to do HIIT or weights is easier than most – I simply am not able to do it. Instead I walk and walk, in ever-increasing circles around my area.

People's bodies and minds do not spring back automatically after major surgery or a major illness. I see this all the time at work, where patients' expectations are that they should be better and back to normal far earlier than they actually are. Even surgeons don't always get this right. They may say that there is an average, for example, of six weeks off work but it is actually GPs who see the patients during their recovery and assess who will need more time. I see patients frustrated with fatigue for a few weeks after the flu, patients who are exhausted because of the strain of mental illness, patients who just want to be better, and better quicker. Our bodies need time to heal, to recover, and they do this by rest; we need to let ourselves do that, no matter how hard it may be, and our minds need to rest too. As a society we need to accept this and allow this of ourselves.

While medicine and surgery have advanced as a society, perhaps we have gone backward in expecting everyone and everything to bounce back straight away to pre-illness states. And even if we accept that we don't, once we feel better we then expect to be able to do all we did before straight away, which again we can't – for example, my physical fitness will take a lot of time to build back up. The corollary of this is that actually recovery takes longer; if we don't allow ourselves time to heal and recuperate then getting ourselves back in both mind and body will be much slower. So we must be patient and accept this.

I admit that this patience and acceptance is a struggle currently and yet with my doctor hat on I can see that I am nowhere near my normal self. If the surgeon had not categorically told me not to do clinical sessions for four to six weeks, I would undoubtedly be feeling that I should (which actually I still do feel). The uncertainty of managing working and how much to work with an as-yet-unknown level of fatigue from chemo is unsettling – I want to plan! Yet I am not even at the point of wanting to leave the house, itching to get out; appointments take so long and so much energy, I am very aware that doing more is simply not possible. I am astounded at my lack of headspace and patience, that even reading a book is a bit of a challenge, that concentrating is so difficult, even as I recognize that this means I am not yet recovered. Yet I am frustrated with myself and how slow recovery is; I want to get back to things, I want to do the things I normally do, I want to be me, and I want it now! Which I suppose is a marker of the society we live in, just as much as it is me behaving like a three-year-old!

THURSDAY 6 JUNE

I had my first psychotherapy session today. This is not something that all cancer patients are offered, though various charities do offer support groups. It was something that I felt I needed, a safe space to talk, somewhere to let it all out, an opportunity to go over and over things if that is what I need without boring anyone. This has all been so fast, I know I need time and space in order to process it, so therapy it is! I was a bit nervous actually, which feels silly: it is just talking, no one is making me go and I don't have to keep going. But I know that talking therapy can be quite hard work, that questioning some of your thoughts and beliefs, no matter how unhelpful they may be, can be quite challenging – even the thinking about things which you don't want to think about, can't think about or haven't thought about can be difficult. I know that it can be normal to feel a little worse before feeling better. I also know that I have been plodding on, keeping moving forward, not really allowing myself to think about it, despite the reams I write here, just constantly thinking about moving ahead, what comes next.

In therapy, I started at the beginning, at this new beginning for me, how I was diagnosed and more; soon I found that I couldn't stop talking as I ran through everything that has happened in the last month. She spoke perhaps ten sentences in the 45–50 minutes we had; the rest was all me, talking, talking, like I couldn't stop, like I write, vomiting my words not on to the page where no one can hear but into the room where she was waiting, listening. I struggled to hold eye contact, especially when recounting the bits which upset me more, but the eye contact didn't seem to matter; I knew she was watching and listening. She expected nothing from me and that in itself allowed me to speak. You see, everyone wants something: if they offer support they want it accepted; if they want to gawp, you are expected to be gawped at; if they are more ghoulish and want the graphic details, you are expected to deliver. Even if they offer love, help and acceptance, like my family do, I know that they have an emotional reaction to everything that happens and so I want to protect them, or I feel guilt when I can't. She expected nothing, which helped me give more than I had expected.

Of those maybe ten sentences that I allowed her time to say, there were some that have really stuck, which, thinking rationally, shows that she probably knows her stuff! The first is that a lot has happened and that it will take time to process it all. I know this theoretically but hearing it from a professional allows me to listen properly; she is saying it is OK for me to think about this constantly, it is OK to not be OK. Secondly, that effectively my life has been hijacked by the cancer but that I am still here somewhere underneath and thirdly, and perhaps most importantly right now, that I am not good at "self". I am a giver, and when I think of myself I think "mother, wife, doctor, daughter, sister, school founder/governor, charity ambassador, friend, author, journalist" all in no particular order, bar the mother first. I mentioned guilt and shame quite a few times, guilt that I am putting everyone though this and shame about doing so. Yet all the roles I described are about what I do or a relationship I have, not who I am, not my "self". I am not sure exactly what that means as all those roles are undoubtedly who I am but perhaps that needs to be challenged. Maybe we should think of ourselves in another way, not just by our roles and what we do, but who are we without those things? Right now I am struggling with the need for "self" and feel in a way that my recuperation is selfish. I need to be better not just for me but for everyone else around me. In telling me there is a lack of self, does that start to enable me to feel less guilty?

FRIDAY 7 JUNE

I went up to see the oncologist again today. My case had been discussed at the multidisciplinary team (MDT) meeting and they all agreed I need chemotherapy. The MDT is a meeting where oncologists, surgeons and radiologists review your history and scans and each use their expertise to create a cohesive and the best-informed plan. I went to the people with the experience and knowledge, and now I will take their advice and have decided I will start with the tablets. I can change if needs be but will start with tablets. Decision made. Making the decision is only the first stage though. Now I need some more time to heal and recover but then comes the reality of the chemo. It is daunting.

SATURDAY 8 JUNE

I am clearly very irritable this morning. Everything is annoying me, from the messages I am receiving to the articles in the paper. It is probably fatigue and discomfort and just the slow process of recovery in general. But what people say and don't say is annoying me today!

The very word *cancer* seems to strike fear into people, to the extent that many of them cannot even say it. "I am sorry you are poorly," they say, or "I heard that you are unwell" or other variations, all the time being very careful to avoid the word *cancer*. The word *cancer* never killed anyone – it is just a word. If we called *cancer armchair* or *chocolate* it wouldn't matter – it is a word, and it is the disease and not the word which harms. I understand, of course I do – people are afraid of it because of what the word represents, what they have seen and what is shown on TV, gaunt bald people having chemotherapy, because they know someone who died. I seem to derive a certain dark pleasure from using the word with people who do not: "Sorry you are poorly" leads to me replying, "Yes, cancer is a pain really, isn't it?" Perhaps this is just me being mean or is it that I need to be brave and brazen this out? If I need to be brave then I need to be brave enough to say the word.

It isn't just the word *cancer* that people struggle with – they also struggle with all the terminology around being unwell. Firstly, people talk about cancer as if it were a battle, that you are a fighter, that you are strong, that you will win and beat it. Cancer is not a tactical decision – I am not going to war for land, for power, or for ethical or moral reasons. If it is a war then I have a possibility of losing, which is something I am not prepared to consider right now. No one makes a tactical error in cancer and therefore loses, so words like *fighter* don't seem to fit.

Neither does a word like *survivor* – it also doesn't feel right. Firstly, I haven't survived in general – I have just survived this bit. I didn't fight – I just lay there under a general anaesthetic while a surgeon did all the work. In fact, the whole having of the cancer and getting rid of it seems rather passive. I had it, someone else cut it out, someone else is going to pump me full of cancer poison (how I have explained chemo to the kids) and I just endured and will endure. How can you survive something when you didn't do anything? And if you survived it, how long does that count for? If it comes back are you still surviving? So I have issues with this word too. Perhaps there are no suitable words, so we use these instead?

Then there are the pictures, the images, the emojis being sent to me of an arm being tensed to show the bicep, of Supergirl flying and more. These are all designed, I am sure, to make me feel or tell me that I am powerful and strong. What they make me feel is stupid because I don't feel strong right now. I am tired, I still bloody hurt and I feel rubbish – I don't think that is how Supergirl is supposed to feel.

I don't even like the term "cancer patient" – is that what I am? Didn't they cut the cancer out of me? In fact, as they got it all, I don't even have cancer right now, do I? So how can I be a cancer patient? The chemo is going to try to stop it coming back, and I hate, hate, hate the thought that although they got it all we still need to treat something in case there is something so tiny, so, so tiny it can't even be seen with a microscope, that is still malevolently hiding somewhere. Biding its time, waiting to come and get me, it feels so evil, so malicious and mostly so unsettling. I digress. If I don't have any cancer in me at this precise moment how can I be a cancer patient?

I know why I struggle with this terminology: it is because I don't want to be a cancer patient/fighter/survivor. Cancer has hijacked and taken over so much of my life, I don't want it to take my identity and my name as well. I am still me, wife and mother, daughter, sister, friend, doctor, author and more – I don't want to be just a cancer patient instead. I need to find a way of accepting that cancer and this time in my life are a part of me now, that I am not "just" a cancer patient instead, that I am a cancer patient as well as. This part of my life will be with me forever, but it can be an addition instead of taking over – I'm just not sure how to do that as yet. While I admit that cancer is now part of who I am, whether or not I like it, why can't I just be called by my name?

Today we went to a soft play with the kids, and after lunch and a nap, we went to the library to change the children's books. It might not seem like much but it is the first time since the operation that I have been out and done something which feels ordinary. To manage sitting in the car without the bumps in the road being torture, to participate in the activity, no matter how small, to join in, it seems momentous.

SUNDAY 9 JUNE

I am still so tired. So bone deep, gnawingly, eye-stingingly exhausted, all the time.

Having a general anaesthetic affects how you sleep: it affects your rapid eye movement (REM) sleep and slow-wave sleep (SWS) for up to about seven days after surgery.

REM sleep is the deepest stage of sleep and is characterized by rapid, random eye movements. REM sleep is linked to dreaming and for adults tends to happen four or five times in a night, accounting for about a quarter of the time you are asleep. There are various theories about the role of REM sleep but it is thought to help maintain brain chemistry, stimulate the central nervous system and help with memory. Slow-wave sleep is the deepest part of non REM sleep and again is thought to be related to memory formation. It takes approximately 90 minutes to reach the REM part of a sleep cycle.

In ICU this lack of sleep was far more intense than on a general ward and is known to cause health issues and affect recovery. The anaesthesia they give you in order to do the operation means that your sleep is already disturbed before you add in the myriad of other issues which stop you sleeping after an operation: pain and discomfort (of course you can't sleep if it hurts), not being able to move around as normal in the bed, it is noisy in hospital, you might be hungry if you aren't allowed to eat, you might feel sick, medications such as steroids may keep you awake, and between observations and tests it feels like people don't leave you alone!

There was also no real differentiation between day and night. The lights may have gone lower but they didn't turn off entirely and I could not see a window or the sky to guide me. Without night or day there was just the passing of an indeterminable amount of excessively slow time.

Imagine yourself, lying on a bed, with the blood pressure cuff going up and down every half an hour, machines squeezing your calves left then right constantly, lying in a half sitting position on your back. I am a front sleeper and not a great sleeper at the best of times but this was impossible. There were medications given at regular intervals through the night, and infusers bleeped – it seemed constantly – if the lines blocked or if the bag was finished. Every time it felt like you may drop off you were woken up.

I was prepared, or at least as physically prepared as I could be – I had an eye mask, I had earplugs – but I really tried and I couldn't do it. In ICU I slept a maximum of forty-five minutes at a time, in a few bursts, maybe to a maximum of four and a half hours' sleep, but on average it was more like three hours, and even those three hours were broken. I couldn't really sleep in the day either – the noise and light were even worse – but I would lie on the bed, sometimes listening to the radio and try to at least relax, and again forty-five minutes would be the maximum. Some people manage better than others on little sleep (not me!) but after a big surgery sleep is essential.

Sleep deprivation is torture, really, the combination of sleep deprivation plus the sound of a screaming baby is literally one of the ways that they torture people, which is why I always feel so much for new parents! I have worked weeks of nights at the hospital, I had three newborns and breastfed them after C-sections, but this was sleep deprivation on another scale entirely. It affects your mental health as well as your physical and adds to the trauma of the whole ICU experience – perhaps this is yet another reason why so many patients on ICU are sedated!

Since being home there has been some progress, but I am still struggling to sleep through. How do you sleep on your back? As a front sleeper this is anathema to me – what exactly do you do with your hands and arms? If they are by your sides or over your chest then don't you feel like you are dead and in a coffin?

I have been propping myself up on pillows, rather like I did when I was pregnant. Yesterday I tried turning over for the first time. There was a combination of relief and pain at being on my front, and I awoke forty-five minutes later on my back, or rather twisting to get back to my weight being off my wound, but I am getting there.

I yearn for sleep, the deep, restorative sleep of the good, the innocent or a child. For my body, for my mind and for my patience and tolerance to be restored. I am a grumpy mother right now, with very little tolerance, snapping and then apologizing, and I feel bad about that. I tell the children that it is because I am tired, but really it isn't enough because when they are tired I tell them that it is OK to be tired and feel grumpy but not OK to be rude. If I set boundaries for them, why am I breaking them myself?

All of this leaves me bone-achingly exhausted. Even when my mind is willing – and to be frank, it is not always willing as the fatigue has affected my memory and ability to concentrate – the body will not follow. As I feel a tiny bit better each day, I want to push myself more, to walk further if not faster, to do slightly more. Yet my body simply will not go – it needs to rest and somehow I need to let it.

TUESDAY 11 JUNE

Today I am going hair shopping. I don't seem to be able to write the word *wig* (yes, I know I wrote it just then). Maybe I'll just need a hairpiece to make my hair look thicker. Ben doesn't really understand why I am getting one; it is possible that my hair won't fall out at all. He thinks I should wait and see, in the same way he thinks I should wait about my eyebrows. The side effects include hair thinning rather than complete hair loss but this can range from a little to a lot. Being anaemic, with low iron, which can cause hair thinning on its own, I have two reasons for my hair to become thin. It may be nothing, a little or a lot, I don't know, and while for him it is a reason to wait and see, for me it is a reason to be prepared. This means microblading my eyebrows, which is a semi-permanent tattoo of individual eyebrow hairs (Thursday's painful joy) and purchasing some hair. If I am called to go on TV, or to a function, and my hair is not behaving then ordinarily I would pile it up in a cascade of messy curls, but if it gets really thin this may not be possible. I want to be able to feel confident that I can look OK, be it with scarves (which look more natural with some hair peeking out if possible), or with a wig. I want to feel confident, I want to feel myself, I want to be prepared. And I would like that wig to look like my hair so want to go now before it changes, which can apparently be within the first and second cycle.

Perhaps it shouldn't matter – I am sure we should all accept ourselves for whatever we are and whatever we look like. Firstly we don't, rightly or wrongly, and secondly what we look like, whatever that might be, is part of our identity, part of who we are. Changing our appearance, in whatever way, including a radically different haircut, can change how we feel about ourselves. Our hair, as women, is linked to our femininity – in fact, in some of the major world religions, either all women or married women cover their hair in public to dress modestly, because your hair is part of what constitutes your sexuality. Like most women I have a love–hate, or sometimes a hate–hate, relationship with my hair. It is curly, and frizzy, and needs work to make it straight or curly; curly girls probably want straight hair and straight-haired girls probably want curls at some point! In fact, I have only recently begun to accept that I actually like my curls! The grass is always greener hair wise, or at least it is until it begins to fall out. When it happened after each baby, and my goodness did it happen a lot, my hair got extremely thin and I found it really difficult to deal with. It may not be perfect, but it is mine.

I wouldn't consider myself a high-maintenance woman. I don't wear make-up in my day-to-day life unless I am doing media work or going out out (and sometimes not even then). I don't wear nail varnish unless it is a special occasion. I very occasionally straighten my hair but most of the time wear it in its natural curls. I don't use fake tan, have eyelash extensions or have whatever the current trend is for hair extensions, not that I am judging those who do – I just don't. I don't even dye my hair, but that is a *not yet* as when the greys come I absolutely will do so. Despite all this, I am spending hours this week on my appearance – wigs today, microblading eyebrows in case they fall out on Thursday. It is slightly alien!

Ben may not fully understand why I am doing this, spending time and money preparing for something which may not happen, but I do. It is about a need to exert control wherever I can find it in a situation over which I have absolutely no control at all. At a time when all there is is uncertainty and unanswerable questions, I feel out of control and frightened. Purchasing a wig, or semi-permanently tattooing my eyebrows, is a way of controlling the tiny bit of my life that is still in my power.

◆

Well... that was a slightly bizarre experience, but far less awful than I had imagined!

Every single mannequin bar one had the same face, a resting bitch face, with a hard thin mouth with bright lipstick on it. Every single wig, even if they looked shockingly bad, looked better on a human head than on the mannequins. The only one with a different face had a neck as long as my arm, like a giraffe. The whole effect was surreal, shelf after shelf of mannequins with the same face yet different hairstyles.

The stylist could not have been more kind, more gentle, or more knowledgeable. He recommended a synthetic-fibre wig, for price, and also because they are lighter and less itchy than real-hair wigs. The store carried each style in one colour, but could order them in multiple shades and tones. This makes the experience a bit more difficult: is the colour right and the style wrong, or the style correct and the colour wrong? I found something which would work pretty quickly, which then meant that I could relax; I think if I had been trying on style after style and getting nowhere I would have got upset fast. Though quite plainly I will be sitting at home crying into a wig at some point, when I can't get it on straight, it won't clip in or just looks wonky! The majority of the wigs in the shop were a light brown, or darkish blonde, mid length and straightish, which probably reflects the hair of most of the clientele. I have shortish, curly or wavy hair in a colour I now know to be called "deep chocolate brown" – useful for when the time comes to dye it!

However, I may not need a wig. If my hair is thin but not too patchy, there is an alternative called a hair topper, which sounds far too similar to toupee! It is like a half wig which you clip on top of your real hair which adds volume to your own. If I keep enough of my hair to have a small section of my own at the front round my face then this may well be enough. The topper matches mine in colour but it is not quite curly enough; it looks like my hair on day three after washing it when the curl is straightening out a bit, which I think should be OK. In the photos I sent Ben, he didn't know if I was wearing a wig when I was wearing it, which must be a good sign.

I decided to take the risk and buy the topper, which he cut shorter so it fits in more with my real hair, hoping it will be enough for now. They will order the wavy/curly wig, which they only had in black, in my hair colour so it will be in stock if I decide to buy it. One perk is that you don't need to pay VAT for a wig for medical reasons (don't try cheating this, as they can check with your GP!), and the topper, which I have called my "wiglet", did cost less than I had expected – giving it a pet name seems to help make it feel more friendly!

Of course we tried on other wigs – surely everyone does? I tried more wavy than curly and more curly than wavy. One transformed me into my elder sister, and the curliest one (which they only had in blonde) into Olivia Newton-John minus the leather catsuit at the end of *Grease*. But most made me look like someone else I know, often people I am related to. Slight variations in my hair style and colour, not necessarily too far from my own, plus some shared genes, and I turn into one of my many cousins!

Which brings me to the names — each wig, hair extension, hairpiece or topper in the shop had been given a name to identify them as opposed to a number. Unfortunately this seems rather ridiculous. "Shall we try on Ivanka?" — I don't usually wear people! "Zoya looks wonderful" — who is she? It all feels rather strange but also slightly removed from me as myself, so perhaps the oddity of the situation helps. I have Evana the hairpiece and the wig is Amor — what is not to love!

WEDNESDAY 12 JUNE

Today is one month from my surgery. One month from having my cancer removed. One month post-op, five weeks post-diagnosis — and the longest weeks I have ever experienced. I appreciate that there was life before this, thirty-nine years of it, but it seems like a lifetime ago, distant and removed, and I am not sure how to get back there.

In comparison to how I was a month ago, or even three weeks ago, I am significantly better; I'm not back to normal but I am far, far better than I was. Sure, I am tired, yes, I am still sore, but it's discomfort, not pain. I can walk about thirty minutes or so as opposed to one or two (or initially none) and can function, albeit imperfectly, at home. One month post-op means that I can get back in my car (as advised by my surgeon) and being able to drive means more freedom — it seems to symbolize getting a part of me back. Even if that part is doing the school run or going to hospital!

The length of time after a surgery before you are allowed to drive will of course depend on the type of surgery you have had. For many abdominal or pelvic surgeries you may be advised to wait anywhere from four to eight weeks depending on the extent of the surgery, but if you had a keyhole surgery it may be far less than that. The rule of thumb after abdominal or pelvic surgery is that you need to be well enough to drive and be able to perform an emergency stop comfortably, but please do check with your medical team. If you have had an operation and are not well enough to drive after three months you must inform the DVLA (driver and vehicle licensing agency).

THURSDAY 13 JUNE

My children's games have got rather dark. The littlest was playing with her first cousin over the weekend. "Let's play our mummies are dead," she said – essentially she is working out her fears and anxieties through play. She plays at hospitals and takes away a teddy for a period of time, telling it it can't see her. In playing "dead mummy" she is working out her feelings. But where did the idea of dead mummy come from? I know I haven't said that to her. I said I had to go to hospital but that the doctors would get me better. The middlest asked if I would die at the beginning, or perhaps she has heard people talking but it clearly is something which is concerning her. She has repeatedly asked if boys can get cancer. I replied that they can without realizing at the time that she was asking about her brothers, she then asked if daddies can get cancer, at which point I realized that she was checking who is safe. This time I avoided the question slightly; I don't want to lie to her but I do want to reassure her. I told her that her daddy is fine, that he doesn't have cancer, that he is here to look after her, that there are lots of people who love her and want to help look after her, and that I am getting better too.

The other day the middlest said that he didn't miss me at all when I was in hospital, and that he wouldn't mind if I died, that he would be fine. Some of this is designed to hurt me, to see what reaction I will have – after all, I hurt him by disappearing for a bit, by not being myself, by changing the constancy of his reality, so he wants to hurt me back. I understand this and can suck it up, can absorb it and respond calmly that his feelings are OK and that I missed him. The death one was slightly harder but I didn't react apart from to say that I wasn't going to die, that I was going to have treatment and get better. He was after a reaction but also perhaps trying to protect himself, trying to practise. If he was fine when I wasn't present, when I was in hospital, then maybe he would be fine if I wasn't there at all. I see the cogs moving, I understand them rationally, but emotionally as a parent it is slightly harder to do!

I wonder about the younger two and magical thinking. Magical thinking is a completely normal stage in child development that tends to occur between about the ages of two and seven. It involves the imaginary world of children and the belief in things which perhaps don't exist, the tooth fairy, Father Christmas, but also an idea that they themselves are magical, all-powerful beings. After all, anything is possible in the world of make-believe. Not only is this useful in terms of developing an imagination and creativity, but it can help with sensitivity and be used as a way to work through events. In more psychological terms, it is the belief that they can control external factors by their own thoughts, and this includes believing they are powerful enough to make bad things happen: "I was cross with Mummy because she told me off because I threw my laundry on the floor, so I made the cancer come", "I was angry Mummy went away, so I made her tummy hurt". These ideas, although normal for their age, may also make them feel worry or guilt. I am trying to prepare myself for if and when the questions come. Of course, with my parental paranoia I am then also concerned that they have not yet arrived; are they having those feelings and not telling me? The not telling is even worse!

The eldest remains full of questions and concerns. He very clearly feels that he has to look after me and is torn between a desire to not have to be a grown-up and look after me, and the need to protect me. I keep reassuring him that he doesn't need to look after me, or anyone, but it doesn't seem to be sinking in. He wants things to remain the same, his routine to be unchanged, and gets anxious when things have to move around, even when dinner time is a few minutes late. He is already going through a period of change, having just done his Year 6 SATs, and will transition to secondary school in the middle of my chemotherapy. This is a significant change in any child's life and he is going to do it with additional stressors.

I am so sorry. Yet that sentence doesn't seem enough. Nor have I said it to the children, even when they say it isn't fair. I agree with them, it isn't fair, and say that I am sorry it is happening but not that I am sorry. I don't want them to have to feel that they have to say to me that they forgive me, or that it is OK. It isn't. And despite the words seeming so trite, simple and inadequate, I really am so, so sorry that I have done this to you. Not on purpose, but my fault. I love you, I am sorry.

FRIDAY 14 JUNE

The roller coaster strikes again and today I am on a downward stretch. Since yesterday I have been feeling really feverish. I saw the GP and had some blood tests and then got sent back to the hospital. Up and down we go, two steps forward, then something else rears its head to worry about. So back to hospital, where the nurses all greet me as they now all know me and the clerking doctor already knows most of my history.

I have pneumonia. I had started coughing the day before but only a bit and presumed it was a virus from the kids. On ICU I had a scan that showed that the bottom of my lungs were not opening, which is almost to be expected – sitting half propped up in bed all day without getting up means that you don't open your lungs fully to breathe (which is why you are given breathing exercises, which I did do!). Lungs that don't open fully are more likely to get infected. The youngest asked me recently why I was so tired and I replied that all my energy was going into making my tummy better, that the energy that I used to send to my arms and legs, to my head, to the rest of me, for playing and other things, is all being used to heal my tummy. Only now we know it isn't: it is half going to my tummy but the rest is fighting a pneumonia!

SATURDAY 15 JUNE

This is a bizarre halfway house, half inpatient, half outpatient, up three times a day to the hospital for the antibiotic infusions. The children were all out on play dates and in between infusions two and three my husband and I went to the cinema – slightly strange! Already I feel constantly nauseous, from the taste of the flush through the line, the taste of the infusions and metallic sensation it leaves in the mouth and the effects of the antibiotics themselves. The surgeon and oncologist discussed the situation and came to tell me what I already knew, that chemotherapy will be delayed. I expected this – you can't start something which will affect your immune system while you are also treating an infection. No one wants to go through chemotherapy, it isn't a lifestyle choice, but now I have to have it I really, desperately want it to begin. Starting it ends some of the uncertainty about beginning and side effects; I will be in it, not waiting to get in, so will keep wading on through. It also means that I would be closer to finishing. And finishing chemo means that I hopefully, hopefully will be done with the treatment phase of this cancer. I get it, I understand the reasoning, but that doesn't make it any the less frustrating.

MONDAY 17 JUNE

I still have a fever. I have had an intermittent fever for what feels like forever.

I am frustrated and I don't feel well.

I want to be better. Not better from this whole thing, I appreciate that that is unrealistic — I just would like to be better from the pneumonia. You see, the doctor part of my brain has begun ticking and it needs to be quiet.

When a patient walks in to see you in general practice, they could be asking about anything, anything at all, so you kind of carry the whole of medicine, or rather as much of medicine as you know, ready inside your head. The textbook known to every medical student up and down the land, called *Clinical Medicine* by Kumar and Clark, is open in your head (ask any doctor and they will have heard of it). As your patient begins to speak and tell you their history you narrow it down, to the correct specialty or chapter in the book, and then narrow your differential diagnosis further and further down until hopefully you land on the right answer, or at least come up with a plan to find it. Added to this is Occam's razor, which essentially means that common things are common, or the other commonly used phrase in medicine, which is: "Don't look for zebras when you hear hooves – it is far more likely to be horses." So your blocked nose could be an allergy, or a polyp which could be benign or more rarely malignant, but is most likely to be due to your viral cold.

I have had a fever now for at least a week. I had one while in ICU and then while in hospital and to be honest I then stopped taking my temperature at home. I had one when they thought I had a wound infection and then stopped taking it again. It is entirely possible and indeed likely that I have had one the entire time since the operation, which is four and a half weeks ago now. So my doctor brain starts questioning. How long is it safe to have a fever for? If I have been on antibiotics for seventy-two hours and there is no improvement, maybe we need to change antibiotics, or add something in? Or maybe it is viral and not bacterial, but then again it has been going on too long. Or perhaps it isn't an infection at all and then we have to think what else could be going on.

TUESDAY 18 JUNE

Who knew that convalescence was a full-time job? I am supposed to go back to work for one half morning later this week and am not really sure how to fit it in! Take today: three trips to the hospital for the antibiotic infusion, and an appointment with a consultant. OK, you may say, but currently you have pneumonia. Choose a more average recuperation day: walking, cancer-related administration such as filling in forms for an exemption for prescription payments, or never-ending household administration, writing this diary, being with the children, sleeping, cooking dinner, walking again – it takes all day. Add into this appointments, of which there are many, from physio to meeting with the kids' teachers to update them, the oncologist, blood tests and many more, and recovery is a full-time job! I understand I am slower, I understand that I am managing my writing work, even though it takes more time, but I thought I would have free time and would be watching box sets on Netflix; I can't work out when to do that!

I know I have written that convalescence is a lost art in here before, but I now wonder if some of that is because it feels selfish. I feel guilty for taking this time, that I should be doing something else, that I should be contributing more to home, to work, not just financially but in many ways. I feel that taking time for myself is selfish. This means that I fill the time that I have, trying to ensure that everything that I can do gets done, so all the bills are paid the day they appear through the door, that the laundry is folded straight away, things that wouldn't matter if they waited a day or so but if I can do them I feel I should, immediately. I feel guilt over spending money on myself, and for spending time on myself for a treat, or even just going to lie down when the children are at home. It seems selfish somehow in a time when I already am being so selfish and taking so much from everyone else. I know I have to, I know that these feelings are not helpful, which I suppose is the first step in dealing with them, but they are there.

Is convalescence selfish or essential? The doctor part of my brain says essential, the human and mother part says selfish. I need to align the two. Sometimes it is essential to be selfish.

WEDNESDAY 19 JUNE

Still coming to hospital three times a day for antibiotics. It is like groundhog day. Last week was one month post-op and I celebrated by driving. Today is five weeks and I am spending all my time in the hospital.

THURSDAY 20 JUNE

I am utterly filled with rage, with spite, venom and anger.

My antibiotic infusion which should take about forty-five minutes took three hours today as they had to get a new line in and had to wait for the doctor to do it as I have rubbish veins. I don't want to be a patient patient.

The new line is in my right hand, my dominant side, and it hurts. Nothing like the pain of day one post-op, or even day seven, but those days are gone and it hurts and I cannot do anything because it is in my hand and it hurts. I can't wash my hands after going to the toilet, and to be honest it doesn't even feel like I can wipe myself properly because I am using the wrong hand. I was prodded and poked and poked and stabbed and stabbed again. I don't want to be in pain and I want to be able to use my hand.

I don't want to be told to relax, or to breathe, zone out or just go with the flow. I don't want to calm down. I don't want to be treated like a patient; I don't want to be a patient! I don't want to have to tell the same story over and over and over again to various doctors and nurses. I don't want sympathy or empathy or to be patted, I don't want apologies or "Sorry, this must be tough". I don't want to hear the same news bulletins on the hour every hour as the hospital waiting-room TV is tuned to the same station. Brexit, we're doomed, Tory leadership contest, we're doomed, economy doomed, everything else in the world, doom. I don't want to talk about cancer, or when chemo will start, or how I am. I don't want to be told I am strong, or brave or doing so well.

I don't want to have to contain my emotions to make you or anyone else feel better. You think you could handle it but you can't – you will try to fix it, you will offer solutions or supposedly comforting sayings. Right now I want to strike out with my words and say hurtful things, whether or not I mean them, just to spew some of my ire. I don't want to have to hear your platitudes or pleas for patience, I don't want to behave and make polite conversation. It won't be over soon, when five minutes feels like five hours and I have been doing this for days and made no progress. I don't want to be told to not get annoyed as it doesn't make anything better. I don't want to keep getting up when you keep metaphorically smacking me in the face. I don't want to pull my big girl pants on for the millionth time, slap on a brave face and keep going.

I want to be apoplectic with rage. I want to scream and shout and break plates. I want to lie on the floor and kick my arms and legs like a two-year-old. I want to feel something. Even people telling me that they are praying for me, which I found comforting before, is making me furious. Your prayers aren't working, nothing is working! I am literally pounding the keyboard. I need to get it out.

I don't want to be positive. I have no need to be positive. They cut the cancer out and I am going to have chemotherapy. Being positive is not going to make the tiniest bit of difference right now. Do you honestly think that the cancer cells toddle off to your brain and decide to invade it depending on whether or not you are feeling positive? Does hope make recurrence less likely, or just all the more crushing when it arrives? There is no point in only saying "stay positive". It might be better to say "be hopeful but plan either way", "try to prepare yourself for the next hit – you know it might be coming at some point" – just being positive doesn't change things at all. I can be pragmatic. I can and will keep going but don't expect sunshine and rainbows right now because today I am spewing bile-filled rage which will swallow up all your positivity until you feel despair and broken. (If I were handwriting this, in very tiny, tiny letters, so small you would struggle to read them, after the last sentence I would have written, *Like me*.)

My grandmother owned a clothes factory in the fifties and sixties. She would tell a story of there being a stack of cheap plates at the front of the machine room on a desk. When one of the machinists would get frustrated or annoyed they would be allowed to go and smash plates. When we were growing up my mother was the same – if we were angry or frustrated as teenagers she would tell that story and allow us to go into the passageway by the side of the house and throw and smash old plates. The only proviso was that we had to then clear up the mess, which tempered the joy somewhat! I want the release of smashing plates.

My anger is palpable. I feel it in my stomach, a churning mass, which may of course also be a side effect of the antibiotics, but I have been angry before – I know what it feels like. My nostrils are flared, my eyes narrowed and my mouth is in a sneer. I feel primed, waiting for battle, which obviously I haven't experienced but I do know what it is like to be waiting in A & E for a trauma to arrive, waiting, ready to pounce, already flooded with adrenaline, but right now with nowhere to expend that energy.

I don't even know what will make me feel better. I just ate half a tube of Pringles because these antibiotics make me feel so damn sick. And of course I am taking the anti-emetics – I am not stupid, stop asking! I don't want to emotional eat (and I sometimes do); chocolate is not going to make this better. I don't want a relaxing bath, or a nap or to watch TV. I can't do my sewing because of a tiny frigging tube in my hand which hurts. It is nothing, so why does it hurt so much? I want to be with people, but I am irritated by everything, I want to be alone. Maybe I don't want to feel better as right now I feel energized by this fury.

I want to go on roller coasters with my kids until I scream with a combination of fear and joy. I want to go to the coast and eat fish and chips by the sea with them. I want to go dancing and have a cocktail. I want the endorphin rush of exercise. I want to have dinner with friends and laugh and have amusing, erudite and interesting conversations. I want to work, to feel that I have achieved something, that I have helped someone else. I want to be considered funny, or interesting, or anything other than unwell. I want to feel hungry, to eat and feel satisfied, not eat because I have to. I want to feel tired, from the end of a busy day, and then revived when I wake up.

I want to hold on to this anger because at least anger feels like something tangible. It feels strong, vital, alive and real; it is something other than pragmatism, apathy or despair. Yet even as I wrote the last paragraph sadness is creeping in, sadness that I can't do all these things right now. I have insight, I know what I am saying here, which is that I don't want to be ill any more (and it isn't even the sodding cancer but pneumonia). I am saying that I want to be me. But I don't want to be sad – I want to be bloody angry!

FRIDAY 21 JUNE

Another day, more blood tests, antibiotic drips and appointments.

Most women, and probably most men too, have unfortunately been taught to hate and despise their bodies.

Too fat, too thin, too lumpy, cellulite, not muscly enough, not defined enough, too asymmetrical, breasts too big, breasts too small, legs too chunky, fat calves, cankles, big bum, small bum, flat bum – I could go on and on. I am no different, though I try not to show my children and to talk about bodies in terms of their strengths and being healthy. For me, and I appreciate that my body fits in with social norms, I would like to be 4 inches taller. Before children (and even after the first C-section) my tummy was pretty flat but with each section, as they seem to sew up tighter than before, an overhang develops, which I hate. The scars from my ectopic pregnancy and appendicectomy faded but the section pouch remained, no matter what my weight was.

Now I look like I have been sprayed with a pepper gun: there are five port sites where the camera and tools were inserted into my belly, three cuts of 2 centimetres and two of 1 centimetre, with a 1-centimetre cut where a drain was left in for a few days to drain away any excess blood, so six small scars peppered over my tummy and a 10-centimetre bigger incision on the left side, set at a jaunty angle.

They had planned to go into my section scar but the surgeon didn't think he could see well enough (perhaps due to the overhang!) so had to make a new incision. So my surgery wasn't really keyhole, rather a bit of keyhole and a bit of open, though I don't have a huge zip running straight down the middle of my tummy. Each of these incisions has a row of dots on either side, ranging from a single dot to about a dozen or so, depending on the size of the scar, from the staples. Some of the scars are dimpling in, and the overhang or pouch is greater than ever, especially on the left-hand side.

I am six weeks post-op. These scars will fade and remodel over the next year or so, changing from being red and slightly raised to hopefully flat and faded. But they will remain, as will that blessed pouch. I am yet to get into my normal clothes, many of which are form fitting – I am not sure if they will fit, or look good and I know I do not need another thing to deal with right now.

I worked hard to think about my section scar, to consider it a marker of pride and not shame – this is how I delivered my babies, which I made and grew and fed. I should be proud of this and not ashamed of a pouch. Why should my body shape, which conforms to societal expectations and norms, be the same as that of a twenty-year-old who hasn't been pregnant multiple times, who hasn't grown and delivered three phenomenal children? It shouldn't be, it can't be, and yet society expects, nay demands, that it is and I am no more immune to that pressure than anyone else.

Yet currently I cannot look at these scars and think of them as positive, in the same way that I looked at my section scar. In time I will, because they are positive, they are stupendous, they are revelatory – they are a sign that I had cancer, that it was cut out, and that I will survive and carry on. These scars represent the removal of the cancer; essentially they represent life. However, the media's obsession with the body beautiful, society's misogynistic undercurrent and often women's own self-hatred battles with this overriding concept; without these scars I would

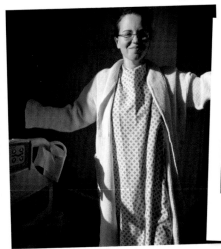

15/5/19

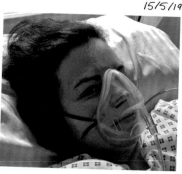

15/5/19

The first pic taken post-surgery after being wheeled into ICU from recovery.

The last pic taken before surgery, sent to my kids to show them Mummy in her hospital gown. Smiling to show them I was okay. Inside I was pretty terrified.

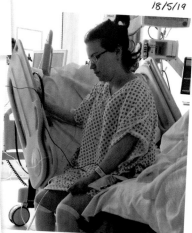

18/5/19

Getting up. I never realized something so seemingly simple could be such a mammoth task.

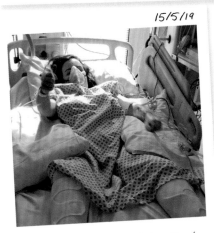

15/5/19

After surgery - at this point the thumbs up were to say I was okay and at that moment I really thought I was, that if this was as bad as it got it was going to be fine.

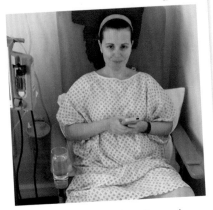

21/5/19

What a difference a few days make - sitting up and smiling! Looking back now I see how exhausted I looked but at the time it was an achievement!

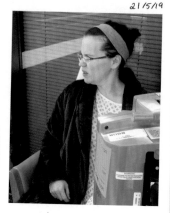

21/5/19

Outside! So incredibly grateful to see the sky.

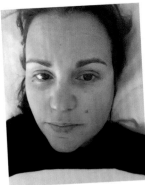

9/6/19

On waking up from a nap at home, recovering.

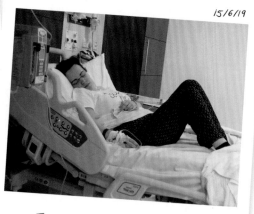

15/6/19

The two steps forward, one (or two, or three) step back path of recovery. Being treated for pneumonia.

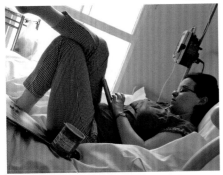

23/6/19

Another day, another hospital visit, more antibiotics.

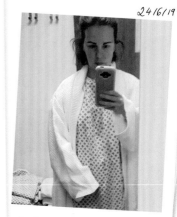

24/6/19

Pre-PET scan, which involves an injection of radioactive tracer. Perhaps I will get superpowers?

14/9/19

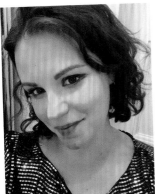

The power of make-up and work, making me feel like myself again!

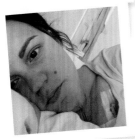

16/9/19

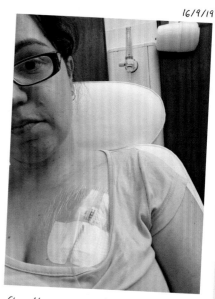

Chemotherapy - hooked up via my port.

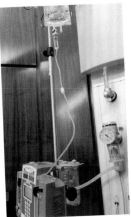

11/12/19

Another day, another drip stand.

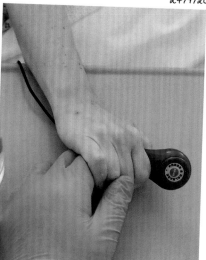

11/12/19

Chemotherapy grenade – a great metaphor, as chemo literally attacks and kills cancer cells.

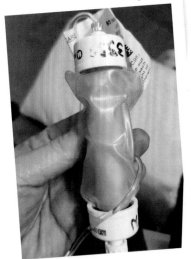

13/12/19

The empty grenade pre-disconnection.

24/9/20

Holding on to what matters post-op, the pain-relief clicker and the hand of someone you love.

be dead, or dying. I should love them, revere them, and yet some part of me still yearns for a flat stomach. How stupid is that? Flat stomach or three children? No question. Three children please. Flat stomach or cancer-free? Without a doubt, cancer-free. Yet I would like the flatter, non-pouchy stomach as well!

Some of this resentfulness toward my body is related to the fact that I don't really understand how, or more importantly why, my body was attacking me from the inside out. It was not my friend, we were no longer a team and currently we are like two strangers learning to get to know each other again. We need to come to new terms, my body and I.

MONDAY 24 JUNE

PET stands for positron emission tomography, and involves small amounts of radioactivity (in the form of radioactive tracers) being injected into you. The radioactivity then spreads through the body and into the cells, and using a special scanner and computer they can then work out which cells are taking up more of the radiation. Active cells take up more tracer, so cancer cells or infection would light up on the scan.

My PET scan was today, and as for most scans or procedures, I was back into a hospital gown – I really am going to have to launch a brand of hospital gowns in better colours or patterns, at least for scans. While I would prefer a gown in a fuschia pink or red, I appreciate that isn't so good for an inpatient as you couldn't see blood on it, but why not for a scan? I could then pretend it is a kaftan! Under the gown went a pair of surgical scrub trousers – size extra large because that is all they had, so they would come up over my bust – and another pair of grippy socks.

I was then taken to a small semi-dark room and the nurse brought in what looked like a small toolbox, or an old-fashioned metal lunch box, lead lined as the radioactive tracer was inside. The tracer is then injected in and you have to lie as still as you can for the next hour to allow the tracer to spread. You can get up for a wee or change position slightly but really you are supposed to lie still. No talking, no TV or radio – the nurse said that the stimulation would make different areas of the brain take up more tracer so the results would be misinterpreted. Instead you just lie in a semi-dark room with nothing but your thoughts for one hour. I am not sure this is the best idea for cancer patients, or any patient who may be a bit worried, as your mind wanders all over the place. Thankfully, I am knackered and so went to sleep for about half of it.

After the prescribed nap, you get up, empty your bladder and lie in a tube which looks like a CT scanner, again completely still for, in my case, about fifteen minutes and then you are done – you just glow in the dark a bit! (Only joking!) The amount of radiation is still pretty small, but the idea of being radioactive for a few hours is very strange!

Then to see the consultant... the scan was normal. Well, not completely normal, but no collection or abscess or anything else. It shows inflammation around the port sites and the surgery, it shows a resolving pneumonia and some inflammation in my left shoulder (which has been hurting on and off incidentally for months) but that was it. No metastases. No other infection. The relief of no spread, the relief of no collection of pus or abscess requiring a procedure, but more frustration and the beginnings of a sense of despair about never being fixed as I still, despite all the antibiotics, have a fever. My white cell count is normal, the markers in my blood for inflammation are low, so what is going on? Now we have to look for something rarer; it is time to look for those zebras.

So on we go. Being a bit of a mystery at the moment but having no infection means that the oncologist might let me start chemo; I mean, he might not if the fever doesn't go, but he might and that is a start! Perhaps I am just unique.

WEDNESDAY 26 JUNE

Six weeks post-op and today I feel better than I have done in the past two weeks, potentially longer. It could be anything from the pneumonia resolving and going away, the phosphate replacement working (a salt in my blood which fell low again and which meant the palpitations came back), or it could be that I just don't feel sick from all the antibiotics I was being given. It is probably a combination of all of those things but who cares. Despite still having a temperature, it is slightly lower and I feel better!

The doctors said it is a four–six week recovery post this operation and they were right. The first ten days were in hospital and the following two weeks at home were very difficult. I was exhausted, I could walk around the block, I hurt and was eating very little on a limited diet. I lay outside and looked at the trees, I lay on my bed and looked at the ceiling and felt no urge to do anything else at all. I did not feel bored or frustrated; in fact, my frustration was that going to appointments meant that I missed my rest!

Between weeks four and six, despite having pneumonia, despite feeling rough as hell and sick as a dog, I also began to feel the stirrings of my body and health returning. Not least in my mind – my mind began to get frustrated with not being able to live life as normal, or at least the new normal, and it is that boredom and frustration that sometimes tell us as doctors that patients are getting better. Not well enough to be doing everything as normal, but better than the completely-content-to-lie-like-a-sausage stage.

Where all my energies before were directed at healing from the surgery, and then to the pneumonia, there was simply nothing left for anything else. While I am still tired and obviously not back to full steam, there is now energy for other things: I can think about going out for a meal, taking the kids to the park (even if I am just sitting watching them); I have the patience and energy to play a board game. Little things, but actually monumental; doing these things is part of who I am, and as my strength returns, I feel myself returning too.

THURSDAY 27 JUNE

I am thankful for the power of make-up, not because I have to cover up, but because I want to look and feel like myself, and for media work that means me in bright red lipstick. The saying is "fake it till you make it" and right now I feel fine but am a pale, exhausted-looking wreck – I need the make-up to make it! There I was on TV and radio with a full face of slap and a dress, looking and feeling like myself, but with a world of turmoil underneath – the TV image and reality do not match but it felt oh so good to remember that I can still do what I do.

Some of my friends keep saying that I am strong. I don't think I am. I just think that something bad happened to me and I am keeping on going. I don't see any other option for me but to keep progressing. This isn't being strong, or being positive – it is being pragmatic and realistic. I can roll into a ball and hide in my bedroom (and sometimes I may need to do that too), or I, like many, many other people, will just keep moving, keep doing what is required to live, to exist. I am in survival mode, the hatches are battened down and I don't have space to deal with anything or anyone else. It isn't about strength – it is about survival.

SATURDAY 29 JUNE

I am a traditional Western doctor, trained in Western medicine, always looking for the evidence base to see what works and what does not. However, I am not against complementary medicine as long as it is just that, complementary and not alternative. You don't get homeopathic vaccines or herbal chemotherapy instead of the vaccines and chemo offered by the NHS, but you can have them in addition if you want! They should complement each other and work together.

The majority of what we would consider medications come from plants, so there are undoubtedly herbal remedies which could work, and various parts of other complementary therapies, such as acupuncture, can be effective for certain conditions including pain. If there is something active in a herb it can work but it can therefore also cause harm, with reports of liver failure with various herbs or interactions with other medications. Aside from active ingredients, there are other parts of these therapies which are unquantifiable, for example that the therapist has time and can talk with you for an hour as opposed to the ten minutes your GP has; that touch is soothing; that lying relaxing for an hour is beneficial, undoubtedly.

All in all I am not closed off to complementary therapies, absolutely not; if they help my patients (or even myself) in whatever way, be it by the talking or the medications, and they can afford it, then go for it. We are all after the same thing: for you to feel better!

I am sore and stiff from weeks of sleeping in unusual positions due to the discomfort from the surgery and various lines, from my core being weakened from being cut into, and because I am not exercising properly. Today I had a massage, nothing too intense, lying on a bed with someone soothing those aches and pains. In doing so, for just an hour I was able to turn off the higher thinking in my brain; all I do is think and think and the stories in my head can be incredibly loud. In having a massage my focus turns inward, into my body and the sensations of the massage itself, and my brain quiets. This has huge value.

MONDAY 1 JULY

I feel good. I feel like myself. Perhaps I would struggle to do a HIIT session but I feel normal, like me, recovered, good to go. A few weeks ago when the oncologist said he didn't think I was quite ready, that I needed to recover more, he was probably right. Now I feel well, despite ongoing low-grade fevers. I feel that my body has healed.

It is quite remarkable really, how resilient we are as humans, that our bodies have an amazing capacity to heal themselves, given enough time to do so. We can survive with quite a lot of bits taken away, we can be cut open and knit ourselves back together, we can lose blood and make more, we can remove part of the gut and reconnect it back together and although it may go on strike for a while, it will start working again. Our bodies are simply phenomenal. I only wish that we could see the wonder in our bodies, for what they do for us, as opposed to only being focused on what they look like. We have an immense capacity for survival, and I am truly grateful to have a body that can heal itself after a huge physical trauma, and a mind that can also heal.

What this means though is that it is time for the chemo to start. I am healed, I am better, come punch me in the face again! Although it is a step into the unknown, it feels like my body would be ready to deal with the next onslaught, which is going to be chemotherapy.

It seems impossible to plan, to predict, to know, about work, about a social life, about being able to pick the kids up from school. We simply do not know what I will be able to do. Currently my "performance status" is zero. This score is out of five: zero means able to get around and do what you want to do, which is currently me; five means you are dead. So a score of one is doing everything but feeling tired, a score of two means you are feeling really quite tired and perhaps doing a bit less than usual, three that you are needing to rest a lot and not managing all your normal activities, and a score of four means you are not able to do much at all due to your fatigue. Apparently I might get to a three. From a zero that seems like quite a deterioration and means that I am worried about planning things: do I plan and cancel, or not plan? All the while there is still no certainty that I will get side effects at all!

TUESDAY 2 JULY

A big day for me today: I went back to work as a GP. Admittedly it was only for half a day (after painful adhesions physio) but still! I was me and people were interested in me as a doctor and not as anything else, which was a relief. It is tiring and I can see that I may well struggle when doing chemo but for the next two months I am planning to do two or three half days on average per week as well as writing and other bits; I think that in combination with the summer holidays, the kids being at home and chemo that may well be enough! If I can manage more then I will reassess after the holidays. But to spend a few hours being the person I was before my diagnosis, being the person that I still am, felt good.

WEDNESDAY 3 JULY

It feels like the chemotherapy tablets should be in a black bottle with a skull and crossbones emblazoned on it. The plain white box with a small neon label saying, *Caution: cytotoxic, handle with care* seems a little underwhelming somehow! I had lots of discussions with the nurses and pharmacist at the clinic about the side effects and what to take for which. As they reeled off the list of side effects over and over, the doubts about my decision to take tablets appeared again. The infusions are easier on the body but are less compatible with normal life, but will I have a normal life for the next six months? Round and round I go in my mind – there are no right answers.

I was given one of those smart cardboard bags with the rope handles, like you get from a posh clothes shop, for all my medication. "Look, you've got shopping bags! Ooh, show me what you got! Oh, just boxes of pills, how disappointing." And I have boxes and boxes. They start you off on a full dose and if needs be decrease it according to any side effects you may have.

I also have a veritable pharmacy of other medications: loperamide for diarrhoea, domperidone for nausea and emergency antibiotics called ciprofloxacin for if they think I have neutropenic sepsis (a medical emergency where you have no white cells to fight infection) and want me to start taking them on my way to the hospital. I have pages of information, lists of phone numbers and details of who to ring, for what and when. Then there are other things which can help with side effects: mouthwashes and ulcer treatments available over the counter and emollients for the sore red hands and feet if they develop. I don't want to wait for them to appear; I would prefer to go and buy them and have them ready and waiting at home, in the same way that as a mother of three children in primary school, there is always a bottle of nit lotion in my house!

It seems so strange that six small, peachy-coloured pills have the potential to wreak havoc on your body! I am not likely to have any side effects for a week or so, yet I am anxious and have to mentally steel myself to take them today. This will get easier, hopefully routine, unless I get horrid side effects, in which case there may be a mental battle each time.

THURSDAY 4 JULY

Today was a pretty ordinary day really – work in the morning, picking kids up, homeworking, preparing supper. It felt good and I felt well in both mind and body. My therapy session was as thought-provoking as ever and I realize that I have been getting irate about lots of stupid little things in the school playground, or that I see on social media. I get annoyed about the superficiality of people, about how vapid some people can be, and yet I realize now that I suppose I am jealous. I am jealous that the most important issue in some other people's lives seems to be make-up, or finding the perfect pair of jeans, while I am dealing with far more weighty matters. Whether or not the perception is the same as reality doesn't matter; it is a feeling of jealousy that other people are not going through this and I am. I don't want to be.

What resources do I have, to make me feel better? What internal workings, or external factors can I use right now to make the situation feel better than it does? The list is short, but we are working on it: my belief in myself, that I will get better, that I will succeed, that this too shall pass; the ability to be in the moment even if it is five minutes at a time, to understand that I only have to survive five minutes, or even one minute at a time, and don't have to think about a whole day, or weeks or months. I don't need to worry about feeling a certain way for three months, I only need to focus on the next five minutes, and I know I can survive five minutes. I can be distracted, by work, by play, by sewing – the repetitive mindful- and mindlessness of it can be distracting. I can ask for company and I can ask to be alone, I can ask to be held. I can smash plates. I can walk, and walk and walk, outside in the fresh air, walk by nature and marvel at the sights and smells (even in London) and feel that there is something much larger than me at play. Right now, that has to be enough.

I continue my tour of complementary therapies after my massage last week and have a session of reflexology. Reflexology is based on the idea that different points on the feet correlate to different points in the body and by gentle massage of the feet one can heal the body, unblock energy and ease stress. With my doctor hat on I can see that if there is something wrong with a joint in the body, or you are hunched over after abdominal surgery, you may walk differently and therefore put differing strains on your feet, leading to muscle tension, which can be eased, though I am not sure of the evidence of healing the whole body through foot massage.

I can also see that it would be relaxing and therefore help with stress and fatigue. I find it soothing and relaxing to be massaged and this essentially was a foot massage, and who doesn't like those? Again, for me it was about getting out of my head and focusing on the sensations in my body, here my feet, which is so relaxing – in fact, I think I may have dozed off slightly.

FRIDAY 5 JULY

Round and round the questions go in my head, about this, about whether or not it is the right decision to try the tablets first, about what comes next, about whether or not I will have side effects, etc. etc. etc. There are no answers to these questions and yet I seek them. I am not used to not knowing the answer. I may not have liked the answers I have come up with for previous problems, I may have struggled with decisions, I may have had to put in the work to produce an answer, but not knowing is not something I really deal with. Even as a GP, if I don't know I find out, I investigate, I liaise with colleagues, I research, I refer on, so even without an answer I still have a plan of what to do next, or who to ask.

Right now planning is difficult as I don't have answers. So I look for them. I ask every doctor, every nurse, the pharmacist about side effects, but asking more people doesn't change the uncertainty around them. I then went to my therapist asking how to deal with the uncertainty, give me an answer for the problem caused by the first question, and again there is no simple answer there to gain acceptance. I cannot turn my head off – my internal monologue is loud, demanding and won't stop questioning.

SATURDAY 6 JULY

I have started following some cancer patients and "survivors" on social media over the last few days. There are some wonderful, inspiring people out there, telling it like it is, or being outliers, showing the world that you can have stage 4 cancer and still run marathons, raise money for charities, raise awareness and more. One of the most famous in terms of bowel cancer is Deborah James, the Bowel Babe, who is utterly phenomenal, with stage 4 bowel cancer at an even younger age than myself, who completes triathlons (which I would and could never do, cancer or no cancer) and does amazing work in the media regarding cancer and so much more.

Some days I feel inspired by them and other days I really struggle to read their posts and blogs, or watch their stories. When they post the amazing things they are doing and achieving, I feel guilty and rubbish for not being able to do much right now; it makes me feel less, and that I should be achieving more. I get cross and say that it isn't a fair representation, that most people four weeks post-op aren't on holiday or doing sports events so it is unfair to those who are recovering as normal to be bombarded with said images (which I am voluntarily looking at by the way!).

When they show the cancer stuff, the realities of chemotherapy, of radiotherapy or cyber knife (a more intense form of radiotherapy), the vomiting, the misery of waiting for scan results, or the exhaustion in general life, it is also too hard to watch. It is too easy to imagine myself in those positions, too easy to identify with their feelings.

There is a fantastic podcast, *You, Me and the Big C* and snippets were posted on social media where Deborah was crying and saying that it wasn't fair. Ordinarily I would listen and think that it wasn't and isn't and sympathize. Now I empathize, and her case is far more serious than mine, but her pain was so acute and real that I could not listen. I cannot allow myself to consider her future as mine – it hurts too much.

Although my feelings for myself are conflicted, I know that they are doing good, lots of good, and I hope to be someone like them when my treatment is done. I have a platform in the media that I can use for good, to raise awareness: I do this for Jo's Trust as their GP ambassador, but with my own story it will undoubtedly be more powerful. I plan to be one of these people. But right now I can't be, which I suppose is another aspect I may be feeling guilty about. It is not that I am ashamed of it – it is just that the whole cancer diagnosis and treatment is a veritable whirlwind without any time to process anything inside your own head and I don't want to do that in any sort of public gaze. It is not a secret, but it is private.

TUESDAY 9 JULY

There is very clearly a doctor's chair in most surgeries or clinics. The bigger chair with the higher back, which might be slightly padded and often is on wheels or spins. You know the one – it is in front of the computer and the patients' chairs are on the side of the desk. It used to be that the patients' chairs were on the opposite side of the desk but the current thinking is that the desk puts a barrier between the patient and doctor and so the patients' chairs are on the side. Very occasionally a patient comes in and sits in the doctor's chair and I never really know what to do in that situation; it isn't that I am being precious about the chair itself, rather I need access to the computer, etc. – that is where the doctor sits! Sometimes, and this happened today, a patient comes in and starts rearranging the furniture, moving their chair right next to mine, which also feels slightly weird somehow. I know this isn't just me; clearly we doctors are quite possessive about our chairs!

I sit in the doctor's chair. That is where I live, where I am comfortable, where I know what my role is. To be fair, I know what the patient role is too – I just don't like it. I do not enjoy sitting in the other chair – it doesn't feel comfortable to me and I don't mean its physical comfort. I don't want to be here and I understand that sounds petulant and childlike but no one wants to be a patient. Of course I have been a patient before, but for the majority of my adult life I have played one role and I much prefer it to the one I am currently in. It isn't about power as such, but about the vulnerability you feel as a patient, and although doctors try to involve you in discussions about your care, you know you are not in control at all.

Even as I sit in the doctor's chair at work it doesn't feel quite normal. Although it works as a distraction and although I am able to focus fully on my patients and their issues, I don't seem to be able to forget that I am also sitting where they are. This may make me more empathetic, or more cautious, or just have a slightly different doctoring style. I don't seem to be able to be just the doctor any more.

I want to sit in the doctor's chair.

WEDNESDAY 10 JULY

Self-care is a very popular buzzword at the moment. Instagram is full of pictures of bubble baths and posts about not feeling guilty about getting your nails done if it makes you feel good. It is about looking after yourself and protecting your mental health, but many of the posts I see seem to forget that it is also about looking after your physical health.

Self-care begins with having enough water and food, a roof over your head, the ability to keep warm, the basic needs for survival. After that, add in looking after your physical and psychological health, taking any medications you need, attending screening, having vaccinations, exercising. When these needs are met then we can begin to focus on the other things you can do to look after yourself, be that taking time out to de-stress and relax with a book, a bath, a walk, a nap, and other things that make you feel good and happy.

My challenge at the moment is to not regard self-care as selfish. I look after myself and my needs, which is the essence of what self-care is, and I feel content and satisfied. Now that my body can do so much more, now I am not forced into submission, I feel guilty about taking the time to do things for myself. My therapist would have a field day and my feelings are probably all linked to my thoughts about self-worth, guilt and blame, but it is a battle for me.

The battle is made easier when a healthcare professional gives me a set of rules for practising self-care – for example, the physiotherapist said I need to walk so I walk and do the exercises I have been set, even if this takes time away from the family. The oncologist said that my skin may become dry so I take the time to moisturise. It is as if I need permission to look after myself. Doing little and resting seems selfish, never mind actively doing something for myself. I tried lying on the swing seat without a book and to be honest it felt uncomfortable, not physically but emotionally! Perhaps this whole process is making me realize how mucked up we all are without the business and chaos of general life butting in and taking up all of our headspace.

FRIDAY 12 JULY

Bleugh. I don't even know how to start today's entry. How do you spell what is essentially a series of groans? Yesterday I went to work and therapy but everything is beginning to be a bit of an effort. I am more tired than usual, and sometimes I feel slightly sick plus today I had abdominal pain, all side effects of the chemotherapy. This one commonly causes diarrhoea, but occasionally constipation, and although it sounds slightly odd to say, a bit of diarrhoea wouldn't go amiss right now! I am up to three sachets of a strong laxative today, my tummy hurts and I am tired. I don't feel well, and if you ask me exactly what that means I don't really know the answer. I feel jet-lagged, or like I'm at the end of a week of night shifts or like I'm coming down with a virus; I just feel non-specifically unwell, and it sucks.

And the knowledge of what is going on is draining. I know that my bone marrow is being suppressed – what is essentially part of what makes my physical essence is being blocked by a medicine I take every day. Chemotherapy aims to get rid of cells which are dividing rapidly, such as cancer cells, but the cells of your bone marrow are dividing quickly too, so they can also be attacked. So I know the damage as well as the benefit that the chemo is wreaking on my body and, just as a battle is being waged in my body, so too is it in my head.

SATURDAY 13 JULY

Today I woke up feeling like myself. With energy, pain-free, no nausea, nothing! The relief is quite intense, not just of the physical symptoms but of the psychological burden that the symptoms would only get worse. This may not be the case – I might not have side effects, or worse side effects, and every day may be different, with some days better than others.

Even though this means I understand there may be ups and downs, it also means that there will be ups. It means that I can continue to be present in the moment, experience whatever it is, but not have the weight of six months of this hanging over my head, that today can be bad but tomorrow can and may well be better. If needs be I can go back to surviving one day, one hour or even five minutes at a time, but needing to survive in such a manner will not be forever.

This may not seem like much, the fact that tomorrow may be better – after all, it may not, and in fact it could be worse – but it gives me back hope and hope is essential for survival, at least for my survival. It gives me possibilities. Not only do I feel physically better today but mentally improved as well, and the two are obviously linked. We as doctors know this and we have all experienced grumpiness when we have a cold, but this is slightly more intense!

SUNDAY 14 JULY

My low-grade fever rumbles on and actually I don't notice a fever under 38 degrees, I am so used to it. I take my temperature regularly as I am concerned that feeling tired or slightly unwell will mean that I won't notice a difference if my fever goes higher, which is a risk for neutropenia (no white blood cells), but today it was my daughter suffering from a fever.

She was a whiny, moaning mess in the morning and got steadily hotter and hotter throughout the day, peaking at 39.3 in between doses of medicine. While this means that I got to watch an epic Wimbledon men's final it also meant that she spent much of the day attached to me, on my lap or napping on me.

When your babies are, well, babies, there is almost constant physical contact between you. I was literally, bodily attached to them for hours each day as I breastfed them, and I mean hours! For every need they had, we had to pick them up and hold them, from changing their nappies to feeding them, to just cuddling and playing with them.

While I may have detached in the literal breastfeeding sense, when they are toddlers there is still a lot of physical contact; it is essential, not just to meet their corporeal needs but for bonding and for comfort. It is also far easier to pick up a screaming toddler who doesn't want to go somewhere than to reason with them!

As your children age, that constant bodily contact diminishes over time. Sure, you still hug, play rough and tumble, wipe faces and kiss grazed knees, but the contact changes. And as a mother I miss it. Perhaps they do too and I don't want to give the impression that we are a stand-offish, no-contact family – we aren't, it is just that it changes from babyhood.

While I hate it when my children are unwell – I am anxious about them and sleep with one and a half ears open (as opposed to the normal motherhood state of sleeping with one ear open) – when they are just a little unwell they give the best cuddles and want nothing more than to snuggle with you on the sofa. As a parent there is a balance to be struck; I don't want them really unwell, but the odd extra afternoon of cuddles is in some ways a bit of a bonus!

WEDNESDAY 17 JULY

The first round of two weeks' chemotherapy is done. Now I have one week off, and as long as my bloods are OK, we start again. Not as bad as I had thought: a few days of feeling pretty pooped in the middle, some constipation and a belly the size it was at six months pregnant from bloating but so far that is it. The side effects are likely to continue into this week but the past few days have been good and I am learning to see the joy in a good day and the wonder of a body that feels like itself, that can go and do what you want it to do and feel well at the same time.

Ordinarily we take this ability for granted; we only moan when we don't feel well, focus on what we don't like about our bodies (and I am just as guilty as anyone else), and don't spend time wondering in amazement at how efficient and wonderful they are when our bodies are working, or even when they are healing or recovering. We should feel joy and gratitude toward ourselves and our bodies, not shame and revulsion! I am learning to feel this relief and appreciate my body on the good days, and to try to remember them if and when the next bad days come.

One cycle down.

There are seven or eight more cycles to come. I am still at the beginning of this journey (can't believe I used the word *journey*), this experience, this time in my life. It is six months in total, and at the start of it, as I still am, it seems like a long way to go. I am still only at the foothills of this mountain, but I am in it now. There may be seven or eight more cycles to go, there may be worse side effects to come, but for today, I am one cycle down. For today, that is enough.

FRIDAY 19 JULY

The side effects are manageable thus far but in addition to the tiredness there are lots of little irritations, dry itchy eyes, dry skin, constipation... any one of these on their own would be manageable but altogether they begin to wear you down a bit. And as ever I can't turn off the doctor, so I treat each side effect as it comes: dry eyes with drops, dry skin with emollients, constipation with laxatives.

I haven't contacted the chemo nurse or the oncologist as I am managing on my own and yet I am not sure if that is correct. If I wasn't a doctor would I be ringing with each new side effect? Should I be managing them myself? As doctors we don't treat ourselves and I am not prescribing myself anything, which would be against General Medical Council guidance. Instead I am using over-the-counter meds and asking my GP for stronger laxatives (which means that the GP checks that my request is reasonable), but essentially I am still in charge of myself.

What this means though is that I am not sure how much I am supposed to manage. If sore dry eyes are a known side effect, how much of that do I have to put up with before they change the dose? If tiredness and feeling rubbish is expected, how much is a reasonable level to deal with or manage before they change something? The answer will be to discuss it with my oncologist but as I am managing I feel I should wait until I see him next week. And yet I don't even know if that is correct either. If I wasn't a doctor would I be ringing for advice now, and even though I am why should I be better able to manage than others? I cannot allow myself to only be a patient and yet cannot also only be a doctor.

SATURDAY 20 JULY

Fifty years since we landed on the moon. Fifty years of innovation in science and medical research. Fifty years ago my outcome and the outcomes of many, many people with cancer would have been very different. Our ever-increasingly sophisticated imaging and screening techniques mean that we pick up cancers earlier and earlier, and when it comes to cancer, time matters: the earlier the better.

The moon landing for me represents much about humanity, about its courage and its urge to explore. It also shows so much about the human body and spirit, and essentially the resilience of both as the impact of being in space and an anti-gravity environment has huge effects on the body. Aside from the issues of no oxygen, extreme temperatures and no water or food sources, we are not meant to live in space; we are designed to live in an environment which has gravity. While you can push out your poo in space, it won't fall off into the toilet bowl like it would at home – you have to help it out! And that is the least of your worries. Despite exercising in space you lose significant muscle mass and bone density among other changes. Yet the experiments performed in space, both on the spaceships and on the astronauts themselves have the potential to continue to make changes in medicine. Fascinating... at least it is if you are a science geek like me!

SUNDAY 21 JULY

My sister-in-law and brother had a baby girl last night and she is adorable and perfect, as all babies are. The pictures make my heart melt and while I am overjoyed for them, there is also a little sadness in there for myself. I love babies, always have done. I am a baby person.

Through the tiredness and emotional mayhem of being postnatal I still adore the really early baby bit, when it is just you and the baby, together in symbiosis. I grew them and nurtured them in my body and then was lucky enough to be able to feed them as well, and there is a unique and relatively short period of time when you and they are essentially one.

I adore that first year, again, despite being knackered: their overwhelming happiness and beaming faces when they see you pick them up after a nap, the gurgling laugh from peek-a-boo and all the other little pleasures that counteract that deep, deep exhaustion! As they get older but are still small I know that I am good at that bit; I can do play dough, I don't mind the mess of glitter (in fact, I love it – it is shiny!!) and I am happy colouring in. In fact, I worry that my parenting skills peaked by the time they were three or four and it is only downhill from there!

I ordinarily solve the issue of one child getting older by simply having another. Well, that sounds awful, doesn't it! I don't mean that it is an issue that my kids are getting older – of course it isn't, it means that they are healthy and well and developing – but I do have a yearning for the baby stage. After my last pregnancy and third C-section, where I had a big haemorrhage and ended up with a general anaesthetic, we decided it was probably best not to have any more. Although the decision was rational, it did not negate my sadness over it emotionally.

This entire situation has been like a reverse pregnancy, with the baby bit coming first, which was me, or maybe the surgical delivery or removal of my cancer, then being unable to do much post-op and drinking milk before weaning back to solid foods, starting to walk again, getting lots of presents, all reminiscent of having a baby! But now with the abdominal bloating, nausea and tiredness, all of which I associate with pregnancy and not chemotherapy, only I now don't have the joy of a baby at the end, rather the joy of finishing chemo!

Every time I go for a procedure or scan, or get medication, I am asked if there is any possibility that I am pregnant and either have to do a pregnancy test or sign that I am not. Chemotherapy and pregnancy do not mix!

I am not pregnant, I have no intention of getting pregnant and indeed I am on contraception to prevent this. I probably could not get pregnant at the moment even if I tried, as the stress my body is under means that it would be less likely to ovulate. My pelvis has had multiple surgeries and another pregnancy would mean yet another one with all the risks that that entails. I know there are no more babies for me, and I know that this is the right choice. Although I am so, so happy for my brother and sister-in-law, I am also sad for me. Knowing rationally that I won't be having more children is one thing, but emotionally, and perhaps even secretly, there is a part of me which still yearns for that stage, especially as the eldest seems to suddenly have got really quite grown up. He is going to secondary school in September and finishing primary school feels like a significant step.

Rightly or wrongly, it feels like cancer has driven the final nail into the baby-making coffin. The door was closed before, but I suppose it was always easier to deal with in my head if it was closed but not locked and bolted. Now it feels triple locked and barred, maybe with a security guard blocking the way as well, and it seems that cancer is to blame for that change.

I am happy for them, and for me and my family at their new arrival, but I will also hold my new niece and breathe in that new baby smell with both love and a little poignancy and sadness for myself. And I think that is OK.

MONDAY 22 JULY

For the first couple of weeks at home I kept having very intrusive thoughts about ICU, to the extent that I was concerned that I would develop post-traumatic stress disorder. I would be doing something else and would be transported back to ICU in my mind, and the same sensations and emotions would envelope me. I would lie in bed waiting to drop off and go over and over in my mind events from that time.

Doctors don't diagnose PTSD straight away because these thoughts, however intrusive they may be, often

go away on their own in time, and the advice is to see a doctor if they are still present after four weeks. Up until then, the thoughts, nightmares and flashbacks are actually part of your brain processing what has happened to you.

Horrible as it may have been, already my time in ICU is fading in my mind. I can bring it back when I think about it and it doesn't diminish how tough it was, but the intrusiveness of the thoughts has gone and it no longer haunts my dreams. Just as my body is healing, so too is my mind.

WEDNESDAY 24 JULY

I saw the oncologist yesterday. My bloods are fine – in fact, they are better than they have been since the operation, despite being on the chemotherapy. My body is holding up well. Essentially he asked me to list my side effects and then simply asked if I was happy and able to continue for another cycle. On we go! Cycle two starts today.

THURSDAY 25 JULY

Today we left for a few days in Scotland. We have two short trips planned in the UK this summer, and although it's not the holiday we planned, it's a holiday nonetheless! We were going to Croatia but I couldn't get travel insurance to cover chemo-related complications and issues and as they are the most likely thing to occur at the moment it did not seem sensible to travel without it. We could have gone to anywhere in the EU (which Croatia is not in), as the EHIC (European Health Insurance Card) means that emergency treatment even related to the chemotherapy would be covered, but Ben was clear that he wanted to stay in the UK. I get it and even agree with him, but am still blaming him entirely! It is reasonable to stay somewhere we know the UK guidelines will be followed, but more importantly actually, that we will be able to communicate and understand what is going on.

As a patient who understands all the medical code which doctors speak in, the thought of not being able to understand anything, or even just partially understand, never mind not being able to explain myself, is extremely daunting. Is this how everyone else feels all the time despite doctors doing their best to translate?

SUNDAY 28 JULY

Edinburgh is a wonderful city, interesting, diverting and we all had a good time. We are now in Crieff, an hour outside Edinburgh, in a huge country hotel with tonnes of activities for the kids and us. It is set in hundreds of acres of land and is utterly, breathtakingly gorgeous. You can see why Scotland is home to tales of the faeries, when every view goes on for miles and ends in mountains, seemingly always in the mist, in varying shades of lilac and grey, overwhelmingly beautiful yet strangely mysterious at the same time.

I find a sense of peace out here, walking in this never-ending countryside, with views that make me gasp around every bend. It is the same feeling that I have in the mountains in winter, of being small and humble and part of something far bigger than me, which seems to put my problems and issues into perspective. We are all part of something far larger than ourselves. While this may seem to be rather troubling for some, for me it brings peace. I can breathe. And breathe and breathe, taking great gulps of the clean, clear air, and feel that here I can be at peace, that perhaps my mind can slow and heal.

MONDAY 29 JULY

Yesterday I did a two-hour high rope course session with the eldest. I love these kinds of things but I haven't done them for a while and he was raring to go. There were multiple courses, each higher and more challenging than the next, with zip wires both connecting platforms to each other and then to the ground. There is nothing to be afraid of – you can't fall off – so the height no longer becomes an issue, rather there is the challenge of completing each obstacle as it comes. Some of them were indeed a challenge! Even if you know you can't fall it still takes some nerve to jump from platform to platform holding on to a rope like Tarzan, not because I was scared to fall, but rather in case I couldn't make it and was stuck swinging on the rope and needing to be rescued! I mean, I never could and still can't do the monkey bars in the playground!

We had a phenomenal time; it was exhilarating, exciting and a wonderful experience for the biggest and I to do together, encouraging each other, looking out for each other and laughing with each other. Two hours of being in the moment, being present, with no other thought in your head bar meeting each challenge and supporting each other. At the end I felt incredibly grateful to have had the opportunity to do this with my son, to be here to do it with him, to be well enough to do it with him.

I may have a bit of a love–hate relationship with the appearance of my belly and my body, but I have rarely been prouder of it than at this time. Approximately ten weeks ago I was in hospital having major surgery. I was in ICU and I could barely put one foot in front of the other. Now I am swinging away, 30 feet in the air, working physically hard and managing it all, not feeling worried about my body, not short of breath or in pain, confident that my body can do this. The resilience of the human body and its capacity to heal and overcome trauma will never cease to amaze me. For my own capacity to do so, and to have this experience today with my son, I am incredibly grateful.

WEDNESDAY 31 JULY

We came home last night and I always get "going-home-itis". Holidays are brilliant – why would you want to go home?

For me, the last five days were a break from cancer and although I was taking my chemotherapy the whole time I felt really good, even if by the end I was more tired than I would usually be. There weren't multiple appointments, reminders about doctors, physio or even therapies to attend, and everything that has defined my life recently just disappeared. It was simply the family and me away, like anyone else, not having to talk about it, not having to deal with it, just having fun, being normal, feeling well, feeling whole.

THURSDAY 1 AUGUST

Today I had a cuddle with my newest niece, and looking at her makes me think, for every new baby and for their parents there is so much hope, so much expectation, so many possibilities. Who knows what challenges she will face and it is both horrible and odd to think that the possibility of illness is already set in her genetic code, though her environment will also influence the expression of those genes and risk of illness.

I look at my own children and feel fear that they may have to go through something like this themselves. I feel guilty enough that they will have to have regular screening from early adulthood, even though it is protective for them, but it is my fault and my illness will mean they will need to go through it. My genes lead to their risk. Actually that isn't true – well, the genes bit is, but perhaps not the fault bit, though it feels that way. I didn't cause the cancer – it is something which happened to me and is separate to me in that way. I need to reframe this thought: the cancer increases their risk, not me. But it still feels like my fault; after all, it is my cancer. I need to learn to separate the two.

SUNDAY 4 AUGUST

I have been feeling good so far this cycle but in the last few days my feet have been hurting, that burning feeling as if I have walked too far, and yesterday they became increasingly painful. To the extent that I looked at them and realized that they were red and that this was probably actually the start of palmar-plantar (or hand-foot) syndrome.

They burned constantly, as if I were running on white-hot sand at the beach to get to cool them off in the sea, but there is no sea, or sand for that matter. Walking barefoot, on carpet in particular, is extremely sore, but so are lots of shoes and the thought of heels is daunting. I think I will be avoiding those! I am in a pair of soft-soled flip-flops and a pair of memory-foam trainers, soft, soft, soft.

Today is much better than yesterday though, and I am finishing cycle two on Tuesday night, and as it is bearable I will keep going. But if this burning symptom becomes cumulative it is a side effect I may struggle with. Pain on every step could really interfere with life, never mind exercise and normal daily activities, which is a little frightening. If it affects my hands too then doing anything, from driving, to cooking, to typing, could be a struggle. The doctor in me doesn't just accept what is happening – it automatically goes to the worst possible point, in order to try to prepare for it. However, I can't prepare for or treat it – I just have to wait and see.

MONDAY 5 AUGUST

I am officially being a spoilt princess. We have gone to Jersey for our family holiday for a week. It is perfectly lovely. Only I don't want to be here.

I want to be on the holiday we were supposed to be on. The one where it would have been hot, hot, hot. Where the sea would have been warm, shallow and mild. Where I could have lain on the beach and watched my kids play in the sand and then swim in the sea and do very little else except eat, and maybe walk around the market and occasionally do a cultural excursion. Where I might have had an afternoon siesta. Where the sun would have baked the heat into my bones, forcing me to relax. Where I would lie on a lilo trailing a foot in the cool sea, floating away into nothingness.

I don't want to be here, even though the coast is beautiful and the sea is bracing and invigorating. I don't want to be here, even though the castles are great and the museums fun.

I just don't want to be here. This isn't really about a holiday at all. In all ways imaginable I don't want to be here, in my life, right now. Cancer is not what I was expecting, not where I thought I would be right now, not in the plan, what I thought would be happening. I was supposed to be all the other things that I am, not this.

I don't think that I have said "It isn't fair" about this situation in general. I have always said it isn't useful, or helpful, and actually I think that life isn't fair. There are no rights or wrongs; good people get sick, bad people get sick, it just happens. But right now, when I want to be on holiday, it feels not fair. And it isn't about the holiday really... the holiday is just a projection of what I am feeling. I don't want this, I don't feel well, it's not fair.

WEDNESDAY 7 AUGUST

I am really struggling. With severe abdominal cramps and pain, constipation, burning feet, exhaustion, and I mean so exhausted that I have to rest my head on the table at lunchtime – literally holding my head up is too much work. I also seem to be short of breath and my heart is racing after I climb to the top of a flight of stairs. It is hard to be away and feel this unwell, and be in this much pain. I want my own bed, my own toilet, just to be left alone. This isn't possible right now; the kids want and need fun on holiday and so I forced myself around a castle. The second cycle of chemo finished last night – this should get better.

FRIDAY 9 AUGUST

It didn't get better – I just felt worse and worse and was in more and more pain. This morning I rang the oncology team;

in hindsight I should have done this earlier and unfortunately the advice was to go to A & E for bloods and an X-ray to check whether or not I had bowel obstruction.

Obstruction is when something obstructs your bowel and nothing gets past, not stool, not liquid, not wind. This leads to extreme pain, abdominal swelling and then nausea and vomiting and requires surgery to remove the blockage. I was almost obstructed before my surgery, and had I been I would have had emergency surgery and would have been much more likely to need a stoma.

I cannot turn off the voice of an extremely scary professor of surgery when I was in medical school who would bellow at us: "What are the top three causes of obstruction?" We would go around in turn, listing the various causes of abdominal obstruction, and he would yell, "No", "Wrong", "Incorrect, imbecile"! He was the old-school humiliate-to-teach kind of a surgeon. I hear his voice yelling in my head: "The top three causes of obstruction are adhesions, adhesions, adhesions!" So much so that I tell that story when I teach about obstruction, just without the humiliation and yelling. Adhesions are formed by scar tissue sticking together. I have had lots of surgery and formed lots of scar tissue, and now I have had bowel surgery. I am at risk of obstruction.

I was very afraid of needing emergency surgery, away from home and heading off to A & E. Though I have found a perk to being on chemotherapy: you tell the A & E triage nurse that you are on chemo and feel unwell and they rush you through to check for neutropenia (no white cells, leading to a huge risk of overwhelming infection), so there is very little waiting! Thankfully this fear was unfounded and the answer was extreme constipation. Basically I was full of shit, plus the chemo itself causes abdominal pain.

The phosphates (one of the salts) in my blood had also fallen again, which explains the inability to climb the stairs without my heart thumping away. So a load of rocket fuel to unblock my bott and some oral phosphates to correct the levels and then back to the hotel to sit by the pool while my kids play.

I was sad not to join them. When a physiotherapist asked me post-op what my aim was, I always replied, to be well enough and mobile enough to play with my kids in the pool on summer holidays. I haven't achieved that, but I also realize that I can't, though I am doing my best and have to look after myself, and the kids are still having fun. We are all doing the best we can.

SATURDAY 10 AUGUST

This morning, after three doses of oral phosphates, I was back. Normal energy levels, yes, a sore bottom from going to the toilet about twenty times in the past twenty-four hours, but back to being me. Being able to do whatever it is I want to do, or at least to climb the stairs without my heart thumping away far too quickly. Just being me. Our day consisted of a ride on a little tourist train along the coast to see the sights, a museum, a funfair and an ice cream. Normal family holiday time. Normal me. Home in a couple of days – I would say back to reality, but it definitely followed me on holiday this time!

TUESDAY 13 AUGUST

If you would have asked me last week if I was ready to start another cycle I would have responded that I was dreading it. That was last week and now I have recovered I don't feel like that at all. I want those extra per cent, those improved chances, so I will go for it. I suppose this is what the week off in the cycle is for, to allow your body some time to heal before you beat it up again!

The oncologist I saw today was very clear that I had side effects which had really affected not just my quality of life but my ability to function and that the effects were cumulative. Essentially if things were pretty torrid in cycle two they were only going to get worse, not better. I am having this chemo as an extra, not as an essential. They cut the tumour out, I don't have cancer any more, so I am poisoning myself and my body in order to stop something so tiny it cannot be seen, which may or may not be there in the first place. This gives me an extra 3.5 per cent decreased risk of recurrence but it is not the same as someone having chemo in order to shrink their cancer pre surgery; this is adjuvant therapy – extra!

Basically, the doctor said that I don't have to martyr myself to side effects. There is an unwritten rule out there somehow, which states that when you are on chemotherapy you have to feel terrible, look terrible and everything must be terrible. And though you might get burning hands and feet – or nausea, or diarrhoea, or constipation, or whatever – this is something to live with and not tell anyone about.

But actually while doctors can't help with all side effects, they can help with lots of them and if we as patients don't tell them they can't help! As a doctor I feel this acutely. Yet as a patient I don't want to bother them – there must be patients sicker than me – and I can or should soldier on.

Essentially he said that I must not. I must not allow myself to be in severe pain, I must not just tolerate everything. I must allow myself to be the patient and let others make decisions with me, not just alone. One of the things that makes him a good doctor is his ability to judge this about me, to know that I might simply carry on, that I need to hear it is OK not to.

It is just so hard to know where that line is, between something which is irritating or inconvenient but manageable and something which is unmanageable and stops me getting on with what I want to do! As such he has dropped the dose of chemo by about 20 per cent. This is not unusual and is something which we knew might happen. It doesn't mean that it won't work; chemotherapy is a balance between being toxic enough to kill cancer but not so toxic that it kills you! Dropping the dose slightly should mean that the side effects aren't so bad, and if they are I will have to change to the infusion type.

I really wanted to get through the summer on the oral chemo. It is far less disruptive to life and the kids, but this has to be balanced against the side effects, which are also disruptive to life and the kids! I have done six weeks of six months of treatment and this will be the third cycle – get through this and the summer holidays will be over. I am having to learn to be in the present, and not think cycles ahead of myself.

THURSDAY 15 AUGUST

Now is the time for me to start committing crimes.

Well, that didn't sound good, did it?

I am losing my fingerprints. Sounds pretty bonkers but I am and this is something which is known to happen with the specific chemo tablets I am taking, capecitabine. The ends of my fingers are a bit sore, are very dry and slightly red, and the top of the tips are shiny, smooth and swollen, so much that the lines of the fingertips are disappearing! Right now it is just affecting the top of them, but apparently it can affect the entire fingerprint. This can last for a few weeks after stopping the chemo but sometimes they don't come back at all.

You would not have thought that losing your fingertips would make any difference to your life at all. If anything it would make robbing a bank easier! But more and more technology relies on fingerprints, to get into your phone or other tech, and apparently even to get into the USA! How annoying would it be to go all that way and then be turned away because you don't have fingerprints?

Do criminals try to remove their fingerprints? How would you even go about doing that? If you burned them then when they healed would they just come back? Shall I even google "can you remove your fingerprints?" or will it trigger someone to investigate me as a potential criminal? Have I gone too far down this wormhole? Most probably. But if they go entirely and don't come back I need to remember to get a letter from the oncologist as to why, so that I can get into the States. Perhaps in the future I will need a different way of unlocking technology!

FRIDAY 16 AUGUST

Patient: "Ooh, congratulations!"

Me: "On what?"

Patient: "On your baby – your pregnancy. You look great!"

Me: [Slightly uncomfortable laugh.] "Oh, I'm not pregnant!"

Patient: "Sorry… but you look pregnant!"

No, that isn't a baby in there. It isn't even a cancer baby in there, just a lot of chemo bloating and a worse shelf/overhang because of all the surgeries and mainly because I eat Pringles for breakfast when I feel sick and so have gained weight.

I have no energy or headspace to deal with the weight gain right now. Instead, I need to be kind to myself, eat what makes me feel better and I will deal with it afterwards. Because I know there will be an afterwards.

SUNDAY 18 AUGUST

Bowel cancer is the fourth most common cancer in the UK, accounting for 12 per cent of all cancers. It is commoner the older you get, being commonest in those over the age of eighty, and over four out of ten cases (44 per cent) are diagnosed in the over seventy-fives. In my age group, the thirty-five to forty-four-year olds, the incidence is ten in 100,000 people in the UK, or one in 10,000, compared to one in 200 men or about one in 250/300 women aged eighty-five to eighty-nine. The sharp increase in rates begins in the early fifties.

GPs act on a set of referral guidelines as to when to refer a patient to a suspected cancer clinic. This means that the patient will be seen by the hospital within two weeks of the referral being made, with the aim that cancers are detected early and so that treatment can be started early, preferably within eighteen weeks of diagnosis (though that target is being missed up and down the country).

Time matters with cancer. The longer you wait, the more likely it is to spread, even though most cancers are very slow-growing. Once you present to the GP with a breast lump, or a hoarse voice for over three weeks with no obvious infective cause, a suspicious mole, or blood in the urine without an infection or other reason, or many other symptoms, you will be referred on a suspected cancer wait to the hospital.

This of course does not mean that you have cancer, or even that your doctor thinks that you have cancer, merely that you have a symptom or sign which could possibly indicate cancer. The powers that be expect that the vast majority of those that we send will not have cancer, will have something benign, but we send everyone with those particular symptoms so as not to miss any.

Although the National Institute for Health and Care Excellence (NICE) sets the recommended criteria, local clinical commissioning bodies (CCGs) use these as recommendations and so there may be slightly different criteria in different areas. For colorectal cancer the criteria for a two-week wait referral would include at least one of the following:

- Tests show occult (hidden) blood in the stool.
- Aged forty or over with unexplained weight loss and abdominal pain.
- Aged over fifty with unexplained rectal bleeding (so if there is a large haemorrhoid which is bleeding then you probably wouldn't refer).
- Aged over sixty with a change in bowel habit – in some areas this says change to diarrhoea only.
- Aged over sixty with iron deficiency anaemia (which is thought to be from hidden bleeding into the stool).
- Consider a two-week referral for those with a rectal or abdominal mass.
- Consider a suspected cancer referral for adults under fifty with rectal bleeding AND any of the following

symptoms if unexplained: abdominal pain, weight loss, iron deficiency anaemia, change in bowel habit.

Note the "consider" in the last two points there. In many areas these are not on the suspected cancer referral forms; you cannot refer a patient into a suspected cancer clinic with those symptoms. We refer patients with suspicious symptoms outside of the age range but these are generally put down as urgent or non-urgent appointments, meaning that they have to wait. And even if you could refer as a suspected cancer wait, I honestly think that I would not have referred a patient who presented as I did, and this haunts me; not for myself, I have been found, but who am I missing?

I had abdominal/pelvic pain as my symptoms, but no weight loss and I wasn't over forty. I also had a perfectly reasonable explanation for said abdominal pain, the adhesions from my previous surgery – indeed I thought it was that! Now that I don't have pain there I realize that some of the pain was right up in my bottom but at the time it all felt very pelvic. As there was another explanation for my pain I would not have been referred as a suspected cancer wait.

There was the very odd occasion when my stool was maroon in colour but this always occurred after I ate beetroot the day before, so I wouldn't have thought it was blood, and it probably was actually the beetroot, as it only happened after eating it!

I had no change in bowel habit, no weight loss, but my pre-operative blood tests showed that I was slightly anaemic. I had not had a full blood count at my doctor's surgery – I had no reason to ask for one, I wasn't tired, I wasn't losing weight, nothing. Even if they had done one for another reason and it was very slightly anaemic it probably would have been put down to me being a menstruating woman who doesn't eat a huge amount of red meat.

I so, so easily could have been missed. If I were my doctor I would have missed me. This is not because I am a bad doctor, or that my colleagues are not good at their jobs. It is because I did not meet the criteria for a two-week suspected cancer referral wait and my relatively young age (in colorectal cancer terms) means that it simply would not have been on the doctor's radar.

If I would have been missed, who else are we missing? Not just in terms of colorectal cancer, but for any cancer, for patients who do not have classic symptoms, or who do have classic symptoms but not within the cut-off age ranges specified on the referral criteria. Aren't we failing them? But if we referred everyone then hospitals would be overwhelmed and would not cope, meaning that yet other patients will fall through the net. Age matters, symptoms matter, as does having a doctor with an open mind, or a mind which has been trained to be open. Despite all of that, I would have been missed. This does not fill me with fear for myself – in fact, I feel fortunate that my cancer was found. Instead it fills me with dread and anxiety about who else may not fit that referral criteria, but may still have cancer.

WEDNESDAY 21 AUGUST

My feet are on fire. If I call the chemo nurses to tell them it feels like I am giving up. It shouldn't but it does, and some part of me feels I should just push through, just finish this cycle, but I honestly don't know if I can.

I am really hobbling today, but will some Compeed be enough to help? Do other patients feel the same, not knowing how much pain to put up with? The GP in me would say to them, "Just phone. Always phone if you are not sure." I feel that somehow I ought to cope better, or know better when to phone or when not to, and be able to manage my symptoms myself because I have some knowledge.

Right now I know why I don't want to ring them. It is because they will tell me to stop and I don't want to stop. Even if it means changing over to the infusions, which I am prepared to do, stopping halfway through a cycle feels like it wouldn't work in some way. Nonsensical in my rational doctor head, yet overwhelmingly present in my patient head.

SATURDAY 24 AUGUST

Two good days and then a bad – sort of like you have to pay for the good days – and even on those two good days my feet and hands were burning, painful messes. I am getting a bit more prepared, more on it with the constipation and upping the laxatives earlier and earlier, but I know that this is not going to be manageable for much longer. When the side effects become so bad that essentially the disruption they cause may well be worse than the inconvenience of the infusions it is probably time to change.

I am going to see if I can last the last few days of this cycle but if it gets much worse than today I will ring and ask for advice. I think I needed to get to this point before changing, the point where I realize for myself that I can't keep going with this level of side effects, especially knowing that they are cumulative, that it will get worse with each cycle.

SUNDAY 25 AUGUST

We were out today when my husband bumped into an old family friend. "How are you?" my husband asked, and got an entire torrent about this person's health, family and more. Conversation over, my English teacher husband said to me that him asking "How are you?" was a prime example of phatic speech, a phrase I had never heard of, but apparently means conversation with the aim of being sociable rather than to obtain information. Essentially you ask "How are you?", but you really aren't interested in the answer; it is just a way of making conversation.

This is absolutely true with me at the moment; people don't want to know, can't hear it, or I don't really want to tell them, yet they still ask, as something to say, and so I reply "OK", or something equally bland. Sometimes I reply that it is all levels of bad, but really I don't want to engage with everyone and answer the questions.

In fact, "How are you?" is so ingrained that if I ask something similar when at work (even though there is a theory that the doctor should stay silent and allow the patient to speak first), the patients always reply "Fine" or "OK". They often then take it back, or launch into why they came, but sometimes there is a pause, and occasionally I respond with "Well, off you go then!"

The same theory applies when people say to me "Oh you look great!", probably without even looking, or seeing whether or not there may be other signals apart from my face that I might be feeling bad, such as body language. No one would actually say "So sorry, you look terrible", apart from close family, who say it as a way of making me go to bed. Friends or acquaintances aren't going to tell the truth when you look bad, and they aren't going to show how surprised or shocked they are, which also means that you can't believe them when they say you look terrific.

"How are you? You look great!" While they are meant kindly, as a form of social intercourse, sometimes it is so difficult to know what the appropriate response would be, so that you aren't the person launching into their full medical history with someone who doesn't really want to know. So I reply "OK, thanks", yet somehow this seems unsatisfactory too.

MONDAY 26 AUGUST

I have had to stop the chemo due to side effects. Today should be day thirteen out of fourteen of cycle three. Yesterday I woke up with a new rash on my back and buttocks but didn't really think very much of it. Today it is worse and I realized that as this was a new symptom – combined with the red-hot, burning feet, peeling hands and cramping abdominal pain – and perhaps one I wasn't expecting, I should ring the clinic. The plan from the oncologist was to stop the cycle if it was bad and then change to the infusions. So, as expected, the nurse told me to stop the cycle with two days left.

I feel that I have failed at chemo.

Clearly, this is not true. Chemo is not something you can fail at, and while rationally I understand this, emotionally I do not seem to be able to. I had to stop. I couldn't finish. This means, in my illogical emotional mind, I have failed.

Logic and theory have nothing to do with my reasoning; it is all emotional. My doctor head knows that killing patients with chemotherapy is not really an oncologist's plan. I know that feeling awful is not good for you, physically or psychologically. I know that chemotherapy isn't more effective the worse you feel, even though we all assume it must be. After all, if it is poisoning me it must be poisoning any cancer too, right?

The doctor part of me knows that chemo can make you feel terrible, so if I feel terrible I sort of think I mustn't complain, even though I also know that the doctor in me would tell patients to talk to their teams, reduce doses, take meds against side effects or stop. Just as with any patient, my brain is a bit scrambled. I can't take out the emotion. I am tired, I can't think straight. I know this is nonsense, I know, yet I still feel like I have failed. I want those extra per cent, I need those extra per cent.

A doctor friend online replied to my stream of consciousness with the following, which cut through the noise in my head: "Be a patient. You want the best possible chance of survival? So does your oncologist on your behalf. He wants to keep his batting average up. Trust him."

TUESDAY 27 AUGUST

Weirdly I was worried that they wouldn't let me change to the infusions, that they would somehow say I had to stop entirely and I would have struggled with that. I know I keep writing it here but it emphasizes my point: I want what the chemo can give me. I saw the oncologist, who stuck to the agreed plan: we will change to infusions.

I should be in my week off starting tomorrow, so the port (the long-term access line) will go in next week and we will go from there. My feet are on fire, my belly hurts, I am exhausted and need to recover before the next onslaught.

I wanted to get through the summer on the oral chemo, to try to prevent too much disruption for the kids. Essentially I have achieved that, so my mindset has changed from one of failure to one of achievement! It was always a difficult decision to make, between orals with worse side effects but only one trip to hospital every three weeks (as long as you don't get admitted in between!) and forty-eight hours of infusions every two weeks but fewer side effects. Neither option is perfect, or obvious. I wanted to get through summer on tablets – I sort of did – and now it is time to change.

SUNDAY 1 SEPTEMBER

A portacath or subcutaneous port is essentially a small plastic reservoir that sits under the skin with a small tube attached which goes into one of the blood vessels near your heart. There are various alternatives, including a Hickman line, where the tubes stick out of your chest, and a PICC line, which sits in your arm. While both of these lines stick out of your skin, a portacath does not. You may have a scar over the insertion site or even see a small bump under the skin but there are no tubes.

A special needle is used to access the portacath so that the chemo can be pumped in. It basically saves your veins, although sedation is often required so ironically you need a cannula in before the very procedure that you are having because you have no veins!

If you are having chemotherapy that involves a four-, six- or eight-hour infusion every few weeks you may well not need a port, especially if you have good veins. The

> **cannula used to give you that kind of chemotherapy is not in for a long period of time, which means that the veins are likely to be saved and survive till next time.**

My kind of chemotherapy is a forty-eight-hour infusion every two weeks. This means that a cannula would need to be inserted for a prolonged period of time. Never mind the fact that they can be uncomfortable in the hand or elbow, they can make it harder to get on with things and the veins are more likely to be damaged, making it harder and harder to gain access each time. So for me, a port is a sensible choice and it goes in tomorrow.

I want the sedation, all the sedation ideally; I have done too much of this awake. I should have been sedated, or at least drowsy, for the colonoscopy, but I think adrenaline overrode whatever sedation there may have been once I saw the cancer.

I was awake for the CT colonoscopy, which was the scan I had straight after my colonoscopy when the cancer was found, for multiple scans, for the PET scan which I was really anxious about, for the spinal and epidural pre-op, for the ureteric stent removal, for two PICC line insertions. All of these things can be done awake but it is exhausting. Your body doesn't know the difference really between physical and psychological stress – for both of them it wants to sleep, it needs to sleep. Staying still for at least an hour, not freaking out, keeping my game face on all the time is a strain. For tomorrow, I would just like to sleep.

TUESDAY 3 SEPTEMBER

They were kind and generous and I slept through the procedure. I have a vague recollection of some patting on my chest but that is it! I am sore and tired, which is to be expected; there is a cut in my chest! My chemo infusions start tomorrow.

WEDNESDAY 4 SEPTEMBER

Why am I nervous? I have already done this. I have had the oral chemo – which essentially is the same stuff – and coped, and this one is supposed to be easier! Yet I am nervous.

I am writing in the chemo chair in the hospital. The treatment suite is divided into relatively large cubicles but it is obvious which chair is the chemo chair and which is for your visitor. The chemo chair is large, padded and comfy and lies flat if you want it to. It is a chair for someone who is sitting for a long period of time! I go to it immediately; it is obvious it is for me, just like the doctor's chair is at work.

I sit here and am grateful not to be stabbed over and over in search of a vein. The port is easy to access and the needle was already sited from the procedure. Here we go; I am in it now.

FRIDAY 6 SEPTEMBER

Having the port and being connected to the infusion for forty-eight hours has not been bad at all. I thought the chemo would be in a pump type thing, probably about the size of a cassette player, and wondered if it would whirr or make noises. Actually it is a ball, about the size of a big plum, and is filled with the chemo. It doesn't pump but works via continuous pressure, going in slowly at 2 millilitres an hour, but is completely silent. I have a little bumbag circa 1990 and the tubing is all under my clothing. It doesn't interfere with anything I do and seems really quite convenient. The disconnection took just a few minutes and was followed by flushing the port. After that, I was good to go.

SUNDAY 8 SEPTEMBER

What does hospital mean to you? A place of illness, death or a place of birth? A place of loneliness and suffering, or somewhere where you go to get better, to be cured? For many people, even walking into a hospital is a struggle. The smell of the cleaning fluid (or fluids which need cleaning), the palpable worry and sight of people who are unwell can make people feel uncomfortable and stressed. People associate hospital with shock, illness and death and often note that the only time you go into hospital for something good is when a baby is born.

I don't see hospitals that way. I appreciate that my view is skewed by the time I spend working in them but I see hospitals as places of renewal and of hope. We take sick people and make them better, we fix broken limbs, treat infections, cut out cancers and deliver babies. We take the worried, the unwell, and we do everything we can to make them better. We don't always succeed but we work together and do our damnedest, all day, all night to help as much as we can.

We see people at their worst and, often at the same time, at their best. We see families come together to support each other, we see people at their lowest, in emotional and physical pain, and yet we see so much love at the same time.

Perhaps it is my way of coping – from seeing so much death at a relatively young age, and coming to the realization very quickly that there are situations far worse than death, to seeing and being involved in tragedies, disasters and even mistakes – to look for what else is there, apart from pain and loss.

What there is, is love, support and comfort, people coming together to help each other and a team of healthcare professionals doing everything they can. I don't see hospitals as a place of fear – in fact, I feel they are a place of comfort and safety. Going to a hospital never caused anxiety in me; even going into surgery, when I have been nervous as hell, I know that I am in the right place.

FRIDAY 13 SEPTEMBER

Today I tried a new therapy, reflexology with hot stones. The combination of the heat from the stones with the massage was hugely relaxing. As I may have written previously, it isn't about the beliefs behind whatever therapy I have had – it is about anything that gets me out of my head and into my body. Anything that silences my infernal, eternal, internal monologue I find very beneficial. Perhaps it is just the lying there for fifty minutes, warm and snug, perhaps the music helps drown out my thoughts, perhaps it is just that massage is nice. It doesn't really matter, it is relaxing and I felt peaceful and I suppose nurtured. I came home tired and slept for two hours – maybe that is the benefit, that it turns off the mind and relaxes the body so you can sleep and heal.

MONDAY 16 SEPTEMBER

The problem with positivity: "You'll beat it", "You can smash cancer", "Just keep positive and everything will be OK."

Positive, positive, positive. Does it really make a difference?

Yes and no. Being negative can have a significant impact on your mental health and actually on your physical health as well, so the corollary would be that a positive attitude may well help. We know that people going into surgery positively seem to have a better outcome than those who go in negatively.

The issue with the stay positive brigade is that you feel guilty when you aren't positive, or when there isn't good news. That somehow you failed in some way, you weren't positive or cheery enough, which is why your cancer got worse. If you can't "beat it", did you fail in some way? It puts all the onus on the patient, and believe me there is plenty of pressure already!

The persistent, unmovable positivity movement does not allow you to feel bad, and even if you have a curable cancer it doesn't leave space to process the enormity and trauma of the diagnosis and treatment. I can see further issues with positivity, both as a doctor and a patient. Not with positivity in general, but with what you are being positive about. If you have an incurable cancer, if you are living with cancer, on chemo, radiotherapy or immunotherapy and living from scan to scan, it is not a failure to not be positive about a cure. It is realistic and pragmatic and allows you to be positive about something else, about non-progression, about stable scans, about more time.

I have seen families and patients so determined to stay positive about a cure that they are unable to let in the possibility of an alternative. So determined that they cannot allow you to help them forward-plan, for palliative care, for death.

There is always something to be positive about but, when appropriate, we need to be open to change from being hopeful for cure to being hopeful to live with cancer, or for a peaceful, pain-free death. What we are positive about needs to be flexible, it needs to change according to the situation, and family and friends need to be aware of this.

To be intransigently positive about beating cancer doesn't allow other positivity, or even acceptance of alternatives. And those alternatives are real; there are many, many people living with cancer for a period of years and years, and there are many patients who are in the terminal phase and are dying of cancer. Acceptance, pragmatism, determination or even peace is not negativity – it is positivity, but aimed at something other than cure.

TUESDAY 17 SEPTEMBER

Last week I joined a gym. I haven't been a member of a gym since I was pregnant with my eldest, which would be about twelve years ago. After the youngest was born and I recovered from the C-section I found that I was getting all kinds of aches and pains and felt more and more tired so I started exercising and it was a panacea. The aches and pains vanished, I had more energy and it felt good.

Not that I am a sporty person, nor a team sports person, but I found that I could do HIIT training. Although it wasn't pleasurable, rather the opposite, all you ever have to do is forty or forty-five seconds of something and even I can survive forty seconds of burpees!

It often made me so breathless, or required so much coordination, that there was no space to think of anything but what I was doing or how many seconds there were left until I got a few seconds' break. A kind of moving meditation. I didn't look forward to it, but I enjoyed the feeling that came afterwards, the endorphin rush, the feeling great!

I did home HIIT workouts, from YouTube, probably three–four times a week and never ever did the mental battle of whether or not to work out go away. I had the angel and devil on my shoulders, one saying work out, but the other, much louder voice would tell me to rest, that I had already worked out once that week, that there wasn't time, that I hurt, or felt tired. Every single time it was a battle to work out, every single time.

My hospital stay and time spent in bed will have meant significant muscle loss and the aim of the physio training since then has always been to maintain me at whatever level of fitness I was post-op. Which was not a remotely high level – I started off walking about 5 metres at a time! I viewed it as medicine; I walked, I followed the instructions and did the exercises.

Now it is time to go to the gym and it can be intimidating in there, not from the men, but from the gym mums! I know as doctors we talk about the importance of physical activity and exercise, and I was active, just at home, or pounding the streets (brisk walking, not running), but it is different in a gym. I can totally see why patients are intimidated by the people in the gym, with their honed bodies, lifting weights, all seeming to know each other and know what to do! But I have as much right to be there as everyone else; maybe I am going slower, or doing less than them, but I am there, trying to stay healthy.

In fact, viewing the exercise as part of the treatment for the cancer, or to prevent recurrence, means that I have more of a drive than before to exercise. Despite being intimidated, the angel and devil on my shoulders have disappeared. I will work out to stay healthy, in mind, body and spirit. I can belong to a gym too!

WEDNESDAY 18 SEPTEMBER

I was back in the chemo suite today.

Rather oddly, this hasn't bothered me at all this week. Last time I was nervous but the cycle was so much better that I am now not nervous at all. Perhaps I should be as the oncologist has upped the dose from 60 per cent to 75 per cent of a full dose but I am not. I feel accepting of the fact that this is what I do now – not necessarily accepting the whole of the current situation, but of the fact that this is what I am doing right now.

Every two weeks I will be here, and actually for the three or four hours I am here I can do what I want. I can write, meet my copy deadlines with no distractions or pulls from elsewhere. I am not available for work, I am not available to pick up sick kids or anything else; someone else will have to if needs be. I am here, and weirdly that brings its own peace.

I sit, I write, I read, I just be.

Until the nurse comes and shoves a whopping great needle into my port! Last time, when it was inserted during the port-insertion procedure, I was sedated so don't remember. I happened to glance at the needle – it looks like a giant drawing pin but thicker, and to be honest it hurts going in. Five minutes later it is OK; there is an uncomfortable sensation but that is to be expected.

I have been aware of the port the whole time since it was inserted; initially it was very sore and bruised but now that it has healed I am still aware of it, especially where the tubing is – I can feel it. I can't sleep on my front and certain movements of my head pull on it somehow. The nurse said it is normal – it takes a long time for the body to get used to the foreign object inside it. Just knowing it is normal is enough; in my doctor brain I just think of worst-case scenarios – is it blocked or is there a clot? – so knowing it is normal helps!

SUNDAY 22 SEPTEMBER

Oh, my hair. My hair.

It is coming out in clumps, big clumps, huge shower-clogging clumps.

I didn't notice any hair loss with the oral meds, but three days after the last infusion the hair started coming out significantly more than normal. Much more than usual and this cycle it is happening again. It won't all fall out – it may just become much thinner.

I have a lot of hair, thick curly hair, and although other people may not notice the difference now I already certainly do. If it continues at this rate then maybe other people will too. I have prepared: I have my hairpiece, I have scarves and headwraps in various colours, I have practised tying turbans so I don't automatically look like I am in a Russian *shtetl* circa 1910, which is my default look when I cover my head. I have prepared physically as much as possible but I don't think you can prepare emotionally.

I am sort of nervous about covering my head. To do the school run, a meeting, work or see friends with a head covering on seems like such a statement. Some of the school mums will say something, some won't – either way it will be noticed. It feels like covering my head says, *I have cancer and my hair is affected*. People will probably presume I lost all my hair so I feel like a bit of a fraud in that it hasn't all gone, or even mostly gone (I have a lot!).

I have been practising with headbands of increasing width but even that is an announcement; it takes my cancer and treatment from being private, or as private as I can make it, to being out there. I have to get used to it.

Today I wore a scarf for the first time; you can still see my hairline peeking out at the front, which makes a difference, but I am trying. It will make my life easier to not have to worry about my hair, to be able to cover it if needs be, but it feels like a lot right now. This isn't a doctor issue, or a female issue, it is just about feeling like me, looking like me, being me.

MONDAY 23 SEPTEMBER

I keep thinking about the point of this diary and whether or not I am prepared to share it with the world. I started writing for me, for catharsis, as a way of taking the many, many jangled thoughts and voices in my head and sorting them out, on paper, or rather on screen. Yet it could be something more, something to help others, though this is not an easy decision to make.

The diagnosis of cancer, surgery, ICU, chemo, etc. are all pretty traumatic life events and I am a thinker – I can go over and over and over something in my head. Somehow writing it down takes some of it out of my head and begins to unscramble the jumbled-up threads of my thinking. It is for me. I even feel the benefits as I write it now.

I have been very private about my diagnosis, telling friends and family and those who need to know but not everyone. A while ago I discussed this with my psychotherapist, who asked why. I replied that I felt I would be lost if I told everyone. That the very essence of me and all the hats that I wear would disappear under the weight of cancer. I would feel that cancer took me away from me, that it would hijack every area of my being, as it literally tried to take over my body.

I felt that if I told everyone then all I would be would be a cancer patient. However, time has passed and things have changed; the surgery seems to be quite distant in my mind now and there is a level of acceptance that it happened. Oh, I am still plenty angry, and often pretty miserable, but there is an acceptance that cancer is a part of me, not physically, but that it is now part of who I am, that it has changed me, as a person and as a doctor. I will always be someone who has had cancer, I will always be anxious before a scan or scope, that anxiety will always be there. But it is not the sum total of me, it is just a part, and I can see that now; from that point of view maybe it feels less scary to put it out there.

The thought of publishing this diary is still hugely frightening, not for people I don't know to read it, but for those I do. I find it far easier to broadcast to thousands than to a group of twenty. This diary shows all my vulnerabilities, it shows me frightened, it shows me weak, it shows my thoughts and fears, and essentially who I am at my very core, when the paraphernalia of the unimportant and the trappings of life are stripped away.

As a doctor, you are taught by experience not to reveal all of yourself, not to let your patients have complete access to your very being. If you did so, there would quickly be very little of you left and you would burn out emotionally. We see people at their worst, which conversely is often when they are at their very best. We see their fears, their aims, their need to survive, we hear grown men roar with grief and mothers scream out theirs, a sound which we never forget. We see abuse, we see situations worse than death, and we are right in there, battling alongside you, doing all we can. You transfer some of your pain to us, and part of our job is to absorb it, or be with you in it. We, as doctors, have to find ways of coping with this, and some of us do it better than others: mental health issues are rife among doctors as are issues such as addiction.

One of the tools which helps is the wall, the emotional wall that all doctors have, that allows the robot within us to continue to jump up and down on someone's chest, to treat a child abused by a parent with compassion and empathy, to listen to a loved one pour out their grief, to watch babies die despite everything that you are doing for them.

We need the robot to survive, yet we need to be human too. The human creeps in, for every doctor I have ever met, for those of us crying in the toilets after a horrific crash call, in those of us excusing ourselves from the ward round momentarily to take a breath, or to find someone to offload to.

We are all human, but if the human is allowed in too much you will find yourself overwhelmed, burned out and unable to cope. Perhaps doctors need more training, not necessarily in communication skills, or even clinical ones, just in how to look after themselves and their mental health.

My human side is often prevalent, and in general practice there isn't the whole medical team to hide behind, it is just you and the patient, one on one. Sometimes if it is helpful I give a little nugget of information about myself, so that they get that I truly understand what they are going through. Sometimes I cry along with them; when people I love cry I always cry too, I can't help it, but with patients it is different – as they tell me of their pain, in whatever form that takes, I absorb some of it, which is why they feel better afterwards, but sometimes this means I cry along too. I always say something as I don't want the patient to feel bad that I am crying, to feel guilt or shame. So I say something like "Just ignore my leaky eyes" or "Don't worry about me – I am crying because you are crying and I really feel how hard this is for you".

For all my concern that the patient might feel bad that they have induced my tears, actually it seems that they really appreciate them, that they appreciate seeing the humanity in me that makes me cry alongside them. Yet we are taught to not give ourselves, because if we give ourselves to everyone there will be nothing left for us. This is one of the dichotomies and challenges of medicine, to be human, to show emotion, to empathize and sympathize and be with our patients along their journeys, yet be able to protect ourselves at the same time.

To publish this diary as a book would be to show my vulnerabilities, to show who I am and to give up myself. No matter how many people you are surrounded by (and I have lots and lots of people who love me), you walk this walk alone. Every procedure, every test, every scan, every chemo, you are surrounded by healthcare professionals whose sole aim is to look after you, and yet you are completely alone. No one else can experience this with you.

I hope that the humanity and experience this diary shows would help others to at least begin to comprehend what it is that their friends, loved ones, or even themselves are going through. At least an awareness or recognition of that, for many of us, would be enough.

THURSDAY 26 SEPTEMBER

My youngest was looking in the drawer beside my bed for a sticker for her bedtime sticker chart and pulled out three envelopes and asked me what they were. I told her they were envelopes and as she is four she accepted that. What those envelopes contain though is the "just in case" letters which I wrote before my surgery.

After she had gone to bed I opened them. I always knew where I had kept them, but wasn't sure why I did – in fact, I am still not sure exactly why I have. There are three letters, one to my husband, Ben, one to my kids and one to my parents. I read them with tears streaming down my face uncontrollably, all the emotions that I had felt when I wrote them flooding through my brain. I thought I had made some kind of peace with the surgery. In general thinking about it now doesn't fill me with dread or pain or anything really, it is just something that happened, but reading the letters opened the floodgates.

The letter to my parents is one of thanks and apologies. In fact, apologies run through all the letters, apologizing for the pain I may have caused. I didn't cause this cancer but I feel, still feel, that it is my fault for inflicting this trauma on those I love. I know it isn't my fault, it is the cancer's fault, but it is still there. Thanks for everything my parents ever gave me, thanks for my life.

The letter to my kids is full of love, but is essentially a desperate message, trying to force a lifetime of love into one letter. How do you do that? I didn't know then and I don't know now.

The one to my husband is not just about love, or sorrow, but also practical things that suddenly seemed hugely important, to cut veggies for mealtimes, to give fruit for dessert, to continue piano lessons and Scouts, to accept help in whatever form that meant. In a different colour pen as an afterthought I wrote a reminder of the time of year when we see the dentist and optometrist for an eye test.

It is the writing of a mother, trying in just a page or two to express what motherhood means and to try to help him be both parents. Of course no letter can teach you how to be both mother and father – I don't even have the answers to motherhood myself, and so it becomes rather practical and staid – but it is the desperate plea of a mother to "look after my children when I can't". The practical took over as I didn't know how to write the emotional. But still I tried to show that I supported him, that I knew he could do it and that above all else I love him.

How do you tell people that you love them? "I love you" is not enough. Love isn't three words on a piece of paper, or said out loud; it is seen and felt in action through a lifetime. "I love you" means taking you to the dentist, and giving you carrots with dinner; it means taking care of you; it means accepting you, being there for you, listening to you. It is action not words, yet words were all I had, if I had to leave them behind.

SUNDAY 29 SEPTEMBER

I appreciate that this sounds utterly ridiculous but it feels extremely strange to be going through chemo and seeming to avoid side effects at the moment. Not entirely, of course – there is the fatigue and the hair thinning – but in comparison to how things were with the oral capecitabine it feels like virtually nothing, which in itself feels odd, as if I am cheating somehow.

As a GP, I see chemotherapy side effects often, as patients tend to speak to their chemo or oncology nurse for advice, or come to us. The list of side effects that I had is not exhaustive and different chemotherapy regimes will have differing side effects while different people will experience them to varying degrees. But there are hints and tips to help for each one:

- Metallic taste – this wasn't a side effect from my chemo but rather from one of the antibiotics I had for ten days or so for pneumonia. It was utterly revolting and constant, and anything which is constant becomes sort of overpowering and all-encompassing – even water tasted disgusting. Here is what helped: avoiding metal cutlery, chewing gum or mints (I used the sugar-free kind), using spices and herbs more heavily than usual, and lots and lots of tooth brushing. Though sometimes the answer was eating Doritos constantly as this overpowered the metallic taste!

- Dry mouth – or just a yucky feeling. Keep well hydrated and try things like a cube of pineapple to stimulate salivation – this also helps if food tastes different or bland.

- Mouth ulcers – the pineapple above helps a dry mouth, unless you have mouth ulcers, in which case it feels like you are eating battery acid so avoid. Washing your mouth out with a salt-water solution twice a day after tooth brushing can be helpful. An alternative is to use Caphosol oral solution, which contains phosphate and calcium and works to lubricate the oral tissues. This is available over the counter but be warned that it isn't cheap, though it is also available on prescription. Over-the-counter ulcer remedies such as Bonjela and Iglü can also be useful.

- Dry eyes – drops, drops, drops. There are lots of over-the-counter dry eye drops available. Use them regularly, about four times a day, and before bed. Alternatively, use a thicker ointment at night – these work very well, but can make your vision a bit blurry so are better before bed.

- Dry, chapped lips – basically everything that can get dry gets dry! You might also get sores in the corners of your lips. Here anything with lanolin in it helps, so brands like Lanolips, or the nipple cream Lansinoh.

- Diarrhoea – this didn't happen to me but essentially most people on chemo will get either diarrhoea or constipation. The answer to diarrhoea is to keep hydrated, and if prescribed use loperamide medication, but be sure to ring your oncology team as your chemo dose may need adjusting.

- Constipation – keep hydrated, eat plenty of fibre and keep active – it literally shakes things down and gets things moving. Use the meds if you need them; bulking agents such as ispaghula husk (Fybogel, for example) are a natural option. An osmotic laxative can be used to pull water into the stool, such as Movicol or Laxido. These can be really effective and you can adjust the dose as needs be. Start off with one per day but you can increase up to eight sachets a day as needed.

- Nausea – for me this was very mild and occasional, but the answer to this one is often to take the drugs, take all the meds you are offered, and tell them if and when you need more or something else! Non-medication remedies include eating small amounts regularly, to stop hunger worsening the nausea, and remedies such as peppermint and ginger.

- Abdominal pain – cramping pain can be related to diarrhoea or constipation but can be treated with over-the-counter medications which contain hyoscine, such as Buscopan.

- Sore hands and feet – or palmar-plantar syndrome. Moisturize, moisturize and then moisturize again. I have sat with my hands in a pot of cream while watching Netflix and it really does make a difference. Ultimately though, when it got significantly worse, with blistering and severe pain, the answer was to drop the chemo dose and then change to infusions.

- Fatigue – this is more difficult to answer, but you need both rest and to keep moving. Exercise during chemotherapy can help with fatigue and to maintain fitness levels but it is also important to listen to your body and rest when you need to. Even though I am not very good at that – I am much better at advising my patients what to do!

So this is my rundown of what I had and what helped – writing it down will help me remember how to help my patients in the future!

TUESDAY 1 OCTOBER

The past two days we have celebrated Rosh Hashanah, the Jewish New Year.

I am a person of faith, and I am proud of my Judaism, its culture, its traditions and most importantly its belief in the family. I enjoy that the festivals throughout the year bring the family together, to eat whatever the food is related to that festival and to sing the same songs year on year. I like the fact that as I prepare for each festival thousands and thousands of people are doing the same thing, at the same time; I feel connected to them both now and throughout history, as in the song from *Fiddler on the Roof*: "Tradition, tradition!"

I believe in something, in a greater being, in a power who has created the wonder of this world, in nature, in reproduction, the seas and the mountains. I don't believe in an all-powerful being who controls every aspect of our lives; I believe in free will. In fact, as with everything, my beliefs are essentially complicated.

Yet I have seen many people who say they have no faith at all appeal to a god or many gods. When the shit hits the fan, sometimes quite literally, and people are sitting by the bed of a loved one, there is a need to do something. And sometimes that something is to pray. Or if not to pray, to appeal and ask for help.

I have seen people who don't believe pleading and appealing, begging God, whoever or just someone, to help, seen them bargain: "I will do anything, anything you want if you could just..." Whether or not God exists doesn't seem to matter – what matters is that at a time when you feel entirely hopeless and helpless there is something you can do and someone to go to for help.

━━━━━━━━━━━◆━━━━━━━━━━━

At this festival, we wish each other a happy new year, a sweet new year and most often a happy and healthy new year. For me, this year, at every greeting, every meeting in the street, people have shaken my hand, kissed my cheek, looked me in the eye and said that they truly wished me a healthy new year, that this year would be better. I am grateful for their wishes, in the same way that I was and continue to be grateful for all the people of many religions who remember me in their thoughts and prayers.

But in some ways, it feels like pressure, pressure to get better because they wish it so, because they are praying for it, because they want me to. I want to be better, of course I do, yet my own hopes for recovery and health are a big enough burden, and adding other people's hopes and wishes somehow sometimes seems to add to the load. I don't believe that having cancer was my fault. I don't. I didn't smoke or drink, I ate fibre, I was mostly healthy, and I got cancer anyway, and even if I did those things I didn't deserve cancer. Good things happen to good and bad people, and bad things happen to everyone. Yet some part of me does feel it is my fault. I don't understand logically how it is, but emotionally I feel guilt about it, guilt that the cancer has caused so much pain to so many people, that it impacts my children on a day-to-day basis. I understand that it is the cancer's fault, not my fault, but sometimes it feels the same.

I sat in the synagogue and I prayed. I prayed for my children, *Happy, healthy, safe*, a mantra, over and over. And I prayed for myself, *Please, when this is over, let it be over and in the past*. Like those relatives, sitting by the beds of their loved ones appealing for help, I bargained, "I will do whatever you want", "I will be better, do better".

I don't know if having faith is a comfort, as it is purported to be. But I do know that the community is a comfort, that I take comfort from other people praying for me, that perhaps somewhere there is a god or gods who might look down and make it all OK. Please, God, make it all OK... happy, healthy, safe.

WEDNESDAY 2 OCTOBER

Today I was back in the chemo suite. Once all the infusions and flushes were done and I was hooked up to the chemo, I strapped the bumbag around my waist and the nurse passed me the little ball of chemotherapy to put into it. As she did so she said, "Here is your chemo grenade", and indeed that is what it looks like, a hand grenade. The wording and imagery are perfect really. In fact, it isn't even a metaphor – it literally is a grenade, a cancer grenade!

I have not practised any visualizations, though I know that other people do, but for the first time after she used that phrase images have been popping into my mind. Images of a seeker grenade wandering around my body and when it comes across any of those too-small-to-be-seen-even-by-microscope cancer cells, they simply explode or fizz away. A cancer grenade – I like it.

FRIDAY 4 OCTOBER

Today I did a whole press conference before having the chemo grenade removed and I honestly think no one noticed. Make-up is a wonderful thing!

Patients need to tell doctors the truth, not to underplay or exaggerate symptoms, just the truth about their symptoms and how they affect their lives, but I have this terrible, really strong urge to underplay everything and to be "good at chemo". I sort of want to please my oncologist, I need to be perceived as a "good girl", a good patient, but my oncologist would only want me to tell the truth!

There is a definite odd push-pull in my head, a need to be the perfect patient but also a worry that they would stop or drop the chemo if I talk about side effects and therefore that it won't work. Rationally, I know that that isn't the case, that we have to balance giving enough chemotherapy for it to work, but not too much that it becomes toxic to you from side effects, but irrationally I worry! I told the truth anyway, which is that it is mostly completely fine, though my hands and feet are red and I am tired.

This week's dose was at 90 per cent of the maximum and, all being well over the next week (as side effects appear in the days after the treatment), then we will go to 100 per cent next time. And then the big news: five cycles to go, over halfway there! Apparently the three oral cycles of capecitabine are the same as about four cycles of 5FU and I have had three cycles of infusion 5FU, so seven down and five to go! Psychologically this is huge. Five doesn't seem so many at all, even though I know I still have another ten weeks to go (starting two weeks from now as I have just had an infusion) and that it ends mid December, which is how long it was expected to take on the tablets anyway. It feels both big and little – big to be over halfway and little because I still have a way to go. On the downward stretch now!

TUESDAY 8 OCTOBER

Physical contact with another human being is important. I use it all the time in my practice, sometimes without thinking, but often knowingly. I started being more aware of it as a medical student, when a little old lady in a hospital bed was telling me that her husband died many years earlier, that she missed cuddles and that now the only people who touched her were doctors and nurses.

Of course the touch of examination is not the same as a hug, nor is touch which hurts, when we take a blood test or give an injection. Often now I touch a patient's arm or hand when they rest it on the table and are upset as they talk. It is obviously a judgement call about who would be comfortable with that and I think it helps that I am a female, but that touch on the arm when you are telling me your story tells you that I am listening, that I feel your pain. It helps us connect, doctor to patient.

The act of physical contact, hugging, etc. is very real. It releases oxytocin, the feel-good, social connection hormone (also released at orgasm), and makes you feel close to the person you are touching as well as reducing stress levels. It can bring down your blood pressure and reduce anxiety, but ignoring the science behind it, it feels good!

My kids and I cuddle a lot, the youngest climbs into my bed every morning at wake-up time for a few minutes of hugs and the older two often find their way into what they call the snuggle, where they lie with their heads on my chest or shoulders with my arm around them, during reading time at night. The almost-twelve-year-old comes for extra hugs daily; there is a need for physical connection. It says I love you, it says you are safe with me.

There is definitely something therapeutic about touch, and that is probably why people like a massage or other touch-based treatments. Sure, some of it is about the physical release of muscle tension but that is not all. Massage, reflexology, whichever complementary treatment I have had has also been about how touch takes you out of your mind and whatever complicated thought processes you are dealing with – even if it just removes you from the constant list-making and routine thoughts, such as *What am I making the kids for dinner?* and *I need to book the dentist* – and puts you back into your body. It connects you back into your physical space and not just your headspace. It is why we like it so much.

People touch me all the time at the moment and have done for months. During the time in ICU I could identify the nurses by their smells we were in such close contact. They clean you, roll you, put tubes in you. They try to be gentle but I was hurting in ICU and most of the time the touch caused pain. The physio helping you out of bed, the nurses supporting you as you walk – constant touch yet none of it with the healing powers of a hug from someone you love. My family sat with me and when I was too unwell to do anything they held my hand, or stroked my forehead, to let me know I wasn't alone. When I told my mother, that very first day, that I had cancer, she put her arm around me and did not let go while the consultant spoke to me, until I had to go for the next scan, as much for her reassurance as mine. As humans, we touch, we hold each other – it comforts, it heals.

TUESDAY 14 OCTOBER

Today I saw a youngish patient with cancer who had a couple of minor things but essentially needed a little space to talk. Being a GP isn't all about diagnoses, tests and treatments; often it is about a period of time where the floor belongs to the patient and they can just talk. You aren't even expected to offer a solution, as you listening is the treatment. She was railing against the "being strong" message, cross that her friends were saying she was a superhero. I saw myself in her – just like me, she said that she didn't feel strong, certainly not superhero-like, but felt that she had no choice. She felt she had to keep going, keep placing one foot in front of the other; she said she did not feel brave. It was like my own voice was coming out of her mouth.

I replied with complete certainty that she did have a choice. That there is always a choice, the choice to curl up on your bed and wait to die, or less extreme to just stay there because you feel sad, or you don't feel well or you feel tired. That to keep going, to keep trudging through is an active choice that she made, no matter what other urges she may have had or how sick or exhausted she feels. That she keeps going, that she goes to chemo knowing it is going to hurt in all the ways that it can. And that is what true bravery is, keeping going when it hurts, going back when you know what is going to happen to you, and she does that week in week out.

She did have choices, and the one that she made was a positive one, a powerful one and one which should be celebrated. She may not feel strong, but by keeping going she was showing that she is, perhaps stronger and more resilient than she realized. I told her to help her realize this and she seemed to absorb it. Her head came up and she looked almost proud as she began to realize that no matter how rubbish she felt, no matter how little she thought she was achieving in comparison to normal, that she was doing well. She had made a choice. Her choice. It was easy for me to see this for her, and in telling her, as she started to believe it, maybe, just perhaps I could believe it even for a tiny bit for myself.

THURSDAY 16 OCTOBER

This month is breast cancer awareness month and the world has turned pink. Pink ribbons, pink lipsticks, pink everything, all being sold to raise money for breast cancer research and awareness, and lots of celebrities getting involved, all raising awareness and discussing the importance of regularly checking your breasts.

This is wonderful, it truly is, and is estimated to have saved about 130,000 lives since the Estée Lauder campaign with Liz Hurley launched in 1992 and has raised millions of pounds for research.

But I am jealous. Or rather my cancer is jealous that not all cancers get the same level of funding or awareness. Breast cancer has an entire month for awareness, and all five of the gynaecology cancers (cervical, vaginal, vulval, womb and ovarian cancers) share a month. Bowel cancer awareness gets a week and there are multiple cancers that don't get the same level of funding or have an awareness programme at all, perhaps because they are less common. "Think pink" is cute, funny, even sexy as a campaign header; "think brown" (as a reminder to check your stools for blood) is notably less so. In fact, it probably turns people's stomachs a bit, which is indeed part of the problem – we are too embarrassed to look at our own poo. It isn't that I want breast cancer awareness to have less – I want other cancer research programmes to have more!

FRIDAY 18 OCTOBER

Here we go again. This time we are up to 100 per cent of the chemo dose and, to be honest, I am feeling it. Today the chemo infusion finishes but I am simply so tired that it is getting really tough. I saw the chemo specialist nurse during my initial infusions two days ago. She comes and asks about side effects and the truth is that apart from a bit of thinning hair, and even that is getting a bit less, though it doesn't want to hold its curl and isn't behaving, the only other symptom I have is fatigue. Fatigue in a way which I have never experienced before, even after having each baby, in fact even after my surgery. I may not have been able to sleep at those times but sleep was restorative – it made me feel better. Now sleep helps but I never wake up feeling raring to go – I feel I could just sleep and sleep and then sleep some more.

I used to be a bad napper, rarely managed an afternoon sleep (even when the baby slept!), and on the rare occasion

I did, if it was past about four in the afternoon, I wouldn't sleep that night. Now whenever I lie down, at whatever time of the day, I can sleep for forty-five minutes or an hour and a half without any problem at all and then sleep in the night.

Exercise helps – it gives me a boost which will take me through the next five or six hours – but in general I am just utterly exhausted. I am working less than normal, but as the chemo accumulates and I get even more tired than I am, I do wonder if I will be able to continue to manage, and if I don't I wonder what it will do to my mental state.

I keep going because I want you to look behind the cancer and remember that I am still here, in whatever hat I am wearing at that particular time. Take away the work and it feels like you take away a hat and leave chemo in its place.

SATURDAY 19 OCTOBER

It is my birthday. Today I am forty years old.

I want to be four and lie on the floor and have a tantrum. I don't want it to be my birthday. I don't want to be forty and have had cancer. I don't want to reach a landmark while having chemotherapy. The weekend after a treatment cycle is always exhausting and my birthday plans will consist of a nap, and probably shouting at the kids because I am tired.

It isn't even that I think birthdays are so important! Of course I make a big deal for the children but for myself I don't usually bother so much. I like presents, of course –

who doesn't! – and I enjoy the excitement that my kids have for me, but I am not someone who would take the day off for my birthday and I probably wouldn't even tell my colleagues.

But I do like a party. Contrary, aren't I? I like parties: I like to throw them, host them, prepare for them, cook for them, get ready and put my make-up on for them. I enjoy the planning almost as much as the party itself. I throw an annual fireworks party, various gatherings at festivals, birthday parties and family teas.

I would have thrown a party for my fortieth. Not because it is such a big deal, more that it is an excuse to have a party. I didn't because I was worried I wouldn't feel well, that I would be too tired, but mainly because I don't want to be forty on cancer treatment. It doesn't feel like something I want to celebrate. I want to be fabulous and forty, not a forty-year-old having chemotherapy for cancer. I just don't.

I am cross and tired, having had chemo the past two days. I am sulking. I don't feel well enough or want to throw a party on chemo and I don't want a fuss, but I want to be able to have and do those things if I want to. I can't and it sucks.

Forty is supposed to be a milestone – perhaps the entry into middle age or the trigger for a midlife crisis, or maybe that is fifty? I don't know, but it feels significant, to be entering a new decade in my life. A new chapter, with slightly older kids, a career, a life. I didn't see this chapter starting with chemotherapy. I didn't envisage this as part of my life, to be honest, not at any age, but never mind now.

Turning forty with a body that turned against me. I don't want it. I want a party, I want to be celebrated and feted. I worked to be here, I deserve it. I don't want this instead.

MONDAY 21 OCTOBER

It is getting hard here. I am just so tired. I don't feel well.

FRIDAY 25 OCTOBER

She was young and diagnosed with cancer, not bowel cancer, but another form. She sat in my office and poured out her fears. She sits in the patient chair, but that is where I also sit now, despite my bottom physically being on the chair of the doctor. She was saying how she felt entirely alone, despite being surrounded by healthcare professionals and her family. I get it, I always got it, I could always see the huge trauma that a cancer diagnosis is, but here I really and truly understood how she felt, because I have felt it too. Yes, we aren't the same, it isn't the same, and even if it were the same cancer or more we still aren't the same, no two situations are. Yet I understood her in a way that I hadn't understood some of my previous patients before.

What came flooding to the fore in my own mind were the memories and feelings which I still have about my own diagnosis, and I couldn't keep these out. So I told her, the first patient I have told – I told her that I have sat in her chair, had a similar experience to her, that I am still sitting there, that she can and will get through this, that she is not alone. She cried, I cried. Then I worried that I was burdening her but she replied that she was grateful to speak to someone who truly understood. With time it will be easier, not that it is right to tell everyone, but it will be easier to tell without the feeling or worry of transferring some of my emotions too.

The further away this becomes from my current life experience, which right now is in it and not far away at all, the easier it will be to reflect and recollect without it hurting so damn much. Then I will be able to let in the human, to show that I truly understand, but perhaps not feel guilty at the same time.

MONDAY 28 OCTOBER

I remember everything. I have always had a good memory and right now it is both a blessing and a curse. Because I remember it all. I can put myself right back in that bed in ICU and remember the exact words he said at diagnosis. I remember pain, I remember the feeling of helplessness, I remember it all. This means I also remember the good bits, the elation of no bag, the sheer joy and overwhelming relief of no nodes, the family, the love. But I remember it all and it hurts to do so, even the good bits. And people don't really want to hear about it any more. The surgery is done, we are on the home straight now, and they don't want to hear about the past, the hurt. "Yes, but you recovered," they say, "Look how far you've come" or "You are so much better". Of course I am – I get that – but the memory of all that trauma, and the ongoing trauma, is still very present in my mind. Yes it was necessary, yes we got it all, yes I am better, I know, I know all that. But some part of me is still that scared girl, tubes in everywhere, lying on a bed in ICU in a haze of pain. I remember it all.

THURSDAY 31 OCTOBER

In medicine you don't ask a question if you aren't going to act on the answer. If you have an elderly patient who doesn't want treatment, why subject them to a whole barrage of tests? If they know what they want and are able to give consent then it is their call. If I am not going to act on a result, why take the test in the first place?

Take, for example, testing during pregnancy for Down's syndrome. The results of a combination of blood tests and an ultrasound scan let you know the risk of having an affected baby. If your level of risk is higher than a particular level you will be offered an amniocentesis or chorionic villus sampling (CVS) which, although the procedure has a small risk of miscarriage, obtains a genetic sample and gives a definitive result. If you know that you would have an abortion if you had an affected baby, then it is worth doing the test. If you know

that no matter what came up you would keep the baby, then you may decide to not have the test, or decide you want it because it would help you be prepared. Either way, essentially you want to know what you think your decision would be before you take the test. Of course, this is only what you think your decision would be as actually being faced with the reality of having to decide may affect your opinion. When it is real it can change how you feel.

I am seeing the cancer geneticist tomorrow. Whatever genes this cancer may be linked to, I now want to know, so that I can act on the results. I will be offered BRCA testing (BReast CAncer genes 1 and 2, linked to breast and ovarian cancer) as part of this, and if the results come back positive I would have a double mastectomy and breast reconstruction now, or rather when the chemotherapy is finished. I would have my ovaries removed at fifty, or if they advised it earlier I would do that too and start hormone replacement therapy. We aren't having more children, so I don't need the relevant parts from that point of view; it would be hard but I would do it to decrease my risks of cancer in the future.

I know what my answer will be but I am still hugely frightened. I am scared of another big surgery – the last one is still too close for comfort – and I am scared of the pain, the change to my body. I discussed it with my husband and while he was fine about the ovaries he was hesitant about the breasts, and the impact on both of us that removing and replacing them would have. But they are mine, not his. I get to choose, perhaps nervously, with trepidation, but it is my choice and he will back me.

FRIDAY 1 NOVEMBER

The geneticist is a bit mind-bending really. They will go looking for genes which are linked to bowel cancer, to know how often my siblings or kids will need surveillance, and also to see which other cancers it may be linked to. If you have X we take out your ovaries, tubes and womb; if you have Y you need an annual gastroscopy as well as a colonoscopy (so one camera down the top and the other up the bottom, top and tail); and if you have Z we take not just your ovaries, tubes and womb but your breasts as well.

Some part of me wants there to be a reason that this happened, even though I know, I really know, that some stuff is just random and happens just because. Yet another part really wants the tests to be negative as positive means more treatment. Then there is an in-between option. When a geneticist looks at genes they are looking for errors, mutations; if they find one, they then look in the database and see if there is any evidence that people who have that mutation become unwell in some way as well as looking to see if it is evident in the healthy population. If it is seen in the healthy population and not the unwell one then it is a random mutation that does not seem to cause harm.

The geneticist told me that when looking at your genes in up to 10 per cent of cases they find a mutation which is not seen in either the healthy or unhealthy population; this is a mutation of unknown significance. So you can have something and not know if it will cause you harm, and a few years later they check the database again to see if it has come up in other people either well or unwell. Therefore, I might be a yes, you have something, a no, you don't or somewhere in between.

Do you know what is so exhausting? All of it. It isn't just the chemo, it isn't just the physical tiredness – it is everything, going to appointments, for blood tests, chemo meds in and out, the oncologist, geneticist, surgeon. So many people involved, so many appointments. Even the psychotherapy is exhausting, not physically, but it is emotionally draining and I often come out feeling wiped. Every appointment, every hospital or centre I visit is a constant reminder of cancer and chemo. The geneticist has put me back in the world of the unknown, which I don't enjoy (nor the three-week wait for results). Psychologically it is utterly draining.

MONDAY 4 NOVEMBER

Side effects are strange things. Some we accept as necessary and others we don't and change meds for. Even on the infusions, which are so much better than the oral type, it is hard. I told the oncologist I was tired and his reply was "yes". There are then questions about how tired is tired, and various scales to complete, but the answer is: I can function but I also need to nap. So we reduced the dose.

There is a sort of unsaid pressure from other people, and if you continually tell me how strong and great I am for keeping going it gets harder and harder to stop, to decline things, to stay home. I gaily wrote here a few months ago about how few side effects I was having but they are there: very dry eyes; dry, peeling hands and feet (without fingerprints, but also without burning pain). The hair loss has slowed down but my hair is definitely thinner and doesn't seem to hold the curl like before.

The tiredness was constant, in a deep way unlike anything I have experienced before. Yet with the 10 per cent dose reduction, although I am tired, it is much better and weirdly better than it was when I was at 90 per cent but going up. Perhaps I am doing less, or perhaps the gym is helping more – who knows? I'm just grateful to feel less tired!

WEDNESDAY 6 NOVEMBER

I can't get one particular lady out of my head. Last week when I saw the oncologist the waiting room was pretty quiet, and I noticed a woman who looked around my age, sitting with someone who was probably her partner and another person. She was noticeably anxious and then was called to see the doctor. I had my bloods and then sat in the waiting room for an hour for them to be processed before seeing my oncologist, so I was in that room for a while.

She returned about thirty minutes later, crying and really obviously distressed. The professor, who is my oncologist, came into the room to give her some papers and knelt beside her, holding her hand, telling her that she was going to be OK.

I can't get her out of my head because I identify with her. I was her, I am her. I sat in that waiting room anxiously waiting to see the oncologist. I cried in his room, I cried afterwards. I know her pain, her anxiety, her thoughts, her worries. Actually I don't, that is a complete lie – I don't know her feelings, I just think I do. I am projecting all of my feelings that I had at the time, that I still have, on to her. Her distress distressed me; it triggered my memories and feelings and it was uncomfortable.

In a way I am worried about her, someone I have never actually met or been introduced to, someone I will likely never see again, but I think about her – is she OK? This is why I can't attend cancer support groups, or group therapy, though I have been having individual therapy. If I go to group therapy I know I will need to "fix" the other members, to offer advice for symptom control, or what to ask your doctor for, to try to help in some way. It wouldn't necessarily benefit me – rather it could burden me. I feel I would feel responsible for the other members of the group in some way, that I would feel they are "mine", in the same way that I feel my patients are "mine", my responsibility.

I may be wrong, but that is why I don't feel group therapy is for me (even though it is an invaluable support for many people), though individual therapy is just fine.

Seeing that woman and absorbing even a tiny amount of her feelings seems to reinforce that it is the correct decision for me.

SATURDAY 9 NOVEMBER

After my initial weight loss in hospital and the immediate aftermath, I seem to be putting it on steadily. Yes, I am resting more and therefore moving less; yes, I don't have the energy to always make healthy food choices and often rely on a sugar rush to give me a bit of a boost; and yes, I am eating a lot of Pringles for breakfast as there is a constant low-level nausea. Even when I made a real effort to eat healthily, not only did the weight not go down (which I didn't necessarily expect) but it continued to go up.

Last week I bought new trousers in a size up. The oncologist said it is common to gain weight during chemotherapy and that many people gain a few stone over the treatment period. This sort of shifted how I feel about it slightly, allowing me to think of it a little more like pregnancy, a period of time where I will get bigger and then afterwards with effort it will go back. It will take work but it will go back. And maybe, like post-pregnancy, it won't go back entirely, but it feels that it will be something back in my control at some point. That I will have control over my body again, which right now is something I don't feel I have – in many ways, not just related to weight.

WEDNESDAY 13 NOVEMBER

Chemo in, counting down, three cycles to go.

Going to bed.

FRIDAY 15 NOVEMBER

Genetics results day.

I have a mutation in the APC gene which doubles your background risk of developing bowel cancer. To start, that risk was small – between the age of thirty-five and thirty-nine there are approximately ten cases per 100,000 females, compared to about 320 per 100,000 in eighty to eighty-nine-year olds – and doubled it is still only twenty cases per 100,000 females. My particular variant of this gene is not linked to other hereditary polyp-causing conditions, such as a condition named familial adenomatous polyposis (FAP), which is a good thing.

I took the tests because the results don't just impact on me, but on my siblings and my children. When they are adults they will now have to make their own decision whether or not to be tested, just as my siblings have to make the choice now. If they are negative then they have the same risks as everyone else and don't need extra monitoring. If they are positive and don't have symptoms then they will be offered a five-yearly screening. As for me, this means that I have to have annual colonoscopies for five years, which become gradually further and further spaced out. But an annual colonoscopy is manageable.

I then burst out, "But what about the BRCA genes?" Negative, all negative, both 1 and 2. And negative for other genes which are linked to small bowel, stomach and oesophageal cancer. A relief. It felt like a breath of air entering my body and with that came a rush of emotion, not grief, not joy, just relief.

I put the phone down and sat there for a bit, trying to process the information. While cancers are likely to have some genetic component and not be entirely environmental, I still felt sort of cross that my body did this to me. Why did it happen? Because bad things just sometimes happen. Why did it happen? Because sometimes these things do. While the majority of me accepted this, some part of me wanted a reason why. Yet now I have a result I don't think I want to know the reason why because it feels like my fault. My genes, my bowel, my body caused the cancer.

I know this isn't correct. I understand on a rational level that I did not intentionally mutate my genes. But there is no other bowel cancer in the family and no way of knowing whether or not I am the founder mutation, that when the sperm and egg joined together to make me that there was a little mistake made (as happens all the time) to cause this.

They are my genes, yet they impact on those closest to me, those who love me. They are my genes, yet they impact on my children, in many ways that we will never know, but I know about this one and I feel bad about it. I know it isn't my fault, but it feels like it is. I don't know if you ever thought about where "you" are in your body, the bit that makes you you, the bit that vanishes when you die, leaving an empty shell, the soul if you are religiously inclined. I have, and I view "myself" as in my head and my head looks down at my body and feels betrayed.

WEDNESDAY 27 NOVEMBER

I don't want to go to chemo today. There is no real reason – I just don't want to. Just as you begin to feel normal you get the next dose, and yes, I am managing fine, and yes, the fatigue is much better at this 90 per cent dose, but I don't want to go. I have had enough. I want to be done.

I went anyway.

SATURDAY 30 NOVEMBER

It is getting harder. The chemo nurse on Wednesday told me that the last couple of months are the hardest part, due to the build-up in your body. I felt nauseous, which I hadn't felt before, and I am literally so tired I feel sick. I have been in bed for the last three afternoons, which hasn't happened for a while. I know there is only one more to go, but right now I am here, not finished, and it is hard.

WEDNESDAY 4 DECEMBER

This is an odd one and it seems that I must be quite contrary, or rather that emotions are conflicting and complicated. I long for treatment to be over, to return to my life, and yet I worry about it. Cancer survivors often find the end of treatment difficult. You go from being almost constantly surrounded by healthcare professionals, with multiple appointments on a weekly or two-weekly basis, where you are in clinic so often that every receptionist and nurse knows your name, to a follow-up appointment six months, one year or even further apart. They describe feeling anxious about this, and feeling that their support network has vanished. As a GP I have had many patients discuss this with me. The answer to which is just to listen, but also to add in that we, GPs and other healthcare professionals, are always here.

I am worried about the end of treatment, even though we are still a while away from this point. I worry that although I have tried oh so very hard not to let cancer take over everything in my life, that I have had to let it in somewhere and that I won't be the same afterwards. That I won't be able to pick up and return to work fully like I did before, or any of my responsibilities for that matter. There are worries about being able to work, even though I know I have done this before – returned to work after maternity leave where I didn't work at all. This time, at least, I have been working through it.

The truth is that I won't be the same afterwards. This experience has changed me, affected me, and we can't just pretend that everything will be the same afterwards.

SUNDAY 8 DECEMBER

I look at photos of myself and my family at recent family events, my brother-in-law's wedding, my father's seventieth birthday, all in the year before my diagnosis. There I am smiling away, all the time growing a cancer in my belly.

Bowel cancer tends to grow slowly. It starts as a polyp which is benign and then turns cancerous and grows. I could have had the cancer for years before it was found, years in which I went to work, looked after my family, went on holiday, worked out, didn't work out, just lived, lived totally unknowing.

How can that be? How did I not know? And if I didn't know then, then how will I know now?

TUESDAY 10 DECEMBER

I am worried this cancer will come back, which is why I worry about chemo ending, and another big fear inside my head is that I will develop a new bowel cancer. You see, I can do everything I am told and be the perfect patient, have the surgery, endure the chemo, eat healthily and exercise regularly, but I cannot change my genes. My genes double the risk of me developing a bowel cancer and having had bowel cancer already makes no difference.

Once you roll a six on the dice, the next time you roll you have an equal chance of rolling another. It feels like my dice are weighted, and weighted against me. Having had a bowel cancer already doesn't change the genes and doesn't change the increased risk of developing a new one. This is why I will have regular scans and scopes for the rest of my life.

This should alleviate my fear, that knowledge is power, but I cannot be rational. The dice are weighted, weighted against me.

WEDNESDAY 11 DECEMBER

Last one! My last chemo cycle started today and I am a mass of different emotions. Today my feelings are a mixture of elation and relief and also fear, a very real fear, for while I am on treatment I am fighting, I am actively stopping the cancer coming back and when it stops will the spectre rise again? Add to that feeling nauseous and fatigue and it is all quite a lot.

But last one... the beginning of the end of this episode. The end?

FRIDAY 13 DECEMBER

My chemo infusion was removed.

We are done.

My God, I hope we are done.

SATURDAY 14 DECEMBER

Earlier this week when I was with the oncologist talking about recurrence and a new cancer, he blithely said, "Your cancer was low risk. We got it in time – it hadn't spread to the nodes". He didn't mean to belittle my experience, but as doctors, even doctors trained in and dealing with cancer every single day, we don't absorb all the feelings our patients have and we don't experience them. To me, my cancer did not feel low risk, ever.

Having a diagnosis of cancer is a trauma, and doctors need to be better at acknowledging and dealing with the emotions that go with this, low risk or high. We are not taught about putting up emotional walls, or how to listen to patients without absorbing all their pain and grief, and I do not recall one lecture about how to protect yourself while dealing with patients, not one.

I was lucky enough to have a job as a senior houseman in psychiatry and during that process I had a weekly meeting with a consultant psychiatrist to help offload and deal with the issues which had come up that week at work. You do not have to have experience in psychiatry to be a GP, and you definitely don't if you are doing medicine or surgery. I was lucky, in that I was given some skills, but the truth is that most doctors learn this on the job, or don't and burn out emotionally. That isn't good enough, not for doctors and not for patients.

Medical students and junior doctors should be taught about *how* to deal with patients' emotions. So I don't blame any doctor who bats away the comment that belies the trauma underneath, or ignores it: they don't know what to do with it.

THURSDAY 19 DECEMBER

It is strange to think that my course of chemotherapy is over while I am still having symptoms related to it. The corners of my mouth are sore and bleeding and I am deeply tired. Many people want me and need me to be better so aren't interested in the effects I am still experiencing – after all, it is over – but my family and close friends seem to understand that although the infusions may be over, I am still in it and the side effects are still there. But psychologically there are beginning to be glimmers of hope. This is the last one, it won't get worse than this, it can only get better.

WEDNESDAY 25 DECEMBER

We have gone skiing on a family holiday. It has been an aim of mine from the very beginning: to be well enough to ski in December. Whether it was for one hour or all day doesn't matter; it represents so much to me, to be well, to be with my family. It is a full stop, the end of treatment and a break away, coming back to a new start, after treatment, when I can begin again.

THURSDAY 26 DECEMBER

I always find the mountains humbling and almost spiritual. When the sun is shining and their majesty is out there in all its glory, when it looks like God has sprinkled diamonds in the snow in the sunshine. Whoever or whatever made their majesty is bigger than I, and it makes my problems feel smaller. I stood on top of the mountain today and was incredibly, hugely grateful to be there, to be whole and healing. There is a bit of a way to go, but I am here, I am recovering, I feel joy, I am so, so thankful to be alive. I think the guidance for cancer patients should be this: don't give up what you love. Do what you love, just do it a bit less and then have a nap!

FRIDAY 27 DECEMBER

Standing at the top of the mountain yesterday I felt truly alive. Perhaps one needs to reach the point of "Thank God I am alive and here" to allow oneself to think of the alternative option.

Although my cancer may have been treatable, it was caught just in time to make it so; it could so easily have been different. I had pain I ignored for many, many months and it would have been possible to ignore it for longer. I could so easily have been missed by the system, or even by good doctors, as no one thought of or was looking for bowel cancer, myself included.

Time could have passed and the cancer could have spread and perhaps death would have been a possibility. Even just writing that feels scary. The thoughts are there but it is only experiencing the thrill and exhilaration of life that lets me consider the other option.

I will not die of this cancer. Not now. I will be a cancer survivor like so many others. Cancer does not have to always be a death sentence.

TUESDAY 31 DECEMBER

It is the end of a decade and I am sure I am supposed to write something profound about the last decade or even the last year but I don't really want to look back at this last year, at least not yet. As for New Year's resolutions, which don't really work anyway, I have but one: to be healthy and whole. How much of that is in my control is not clear but whatever I can do I will do. I wish the same for my family and loved ones, happy and healthy. It is all that matters really.

SUNDAY 5 JANUARY 2020

Is there an expectation to return to normal? Whatever your normal might have been? I think there is but I can't quite yet see if that expectation is coming from others or from within. Certainly the children want normality back, but for them that is a mummy who has the energy to play and go out and doesn't keep going to hospital.

The truth is, there is no going back. Not to that normal, only to a new one. I am not the same person as the one who didn't have cancer – this was a major trauma, both physically and mentally, both of which leave scars. I am not the same. I am stronger, more resilient, but I also have a renewed respect for the importance of looking after one's body and mind in all the forms that that takes. Philippa 2.0 post-cancer is different. I have more empathy, more understanding. Cancer does not always take away – it can give, and I can see that and its value.

I will find my new normal. It will probably take some time, but there is life after this episode, lots of it, and I intend to appreciate it!

WEDNESDAY 8 JANUARY

For about a week now I have been waking up in the morning and feeling, well, good! Perhaps you don't know how bad you have been feeling until you don't feel it any more? I knew I was tired and felt generally a bit rubbish but I think somehow I had forgotten that that isn't how I usually feel! Yes, I get tired and am probably deconditioned so get tired more easily than normal, but there is a difference in the tiredness – it feels ordinary and not the deep bone-aching fatigue of before.

I feel like I recognize my body for the first time in a long time. I feel I know what my body is telling me, that its signals are ones I recognize from before. I am healing, I will be whole. The body, my body, is tough and, actually, extraordinary in its capacity to heal. This feels really quite momentous; in fact, while I would not recommend being on chemotherapy as enjoyable, coming off it feels brilliant!

MONDAY 13 JANUARY

Feeling good, or actually feeling normal, felt so good it is almost a kind of euphoria. The corners of my mouth aren't splitting open every time I open my mouth to eat, my fingers and toes aren't peeling, my eyes aren't watering from constant dryness, basically I am not parched from top to toe any more. My skin doesn't look dull and even slightly grey. I look more like me. The euphoria couldn't last forever though and yesterday, after a busy weekend, I felt tired by about 5 p.m. Feeling tired though not nauseous with fatigue, but there was still a moment of panic: am I going backward? Is the feeling good over? Am I back to exhaustion? Of course not, it is just normal tiredness, everyone gets tired at the end of a busy week, and between work and three kids, every week is a busy week. I have to remember this is normal.

THURSDAY 16 JANUARY

I write this at 3.49 a.m. I cannot sleep. As I wrote here nine months ago, sleep is often affected by stress.

Today is results day for my scans and as the clock ticks steadily nearer, I begin to feel slightly sick with nerves. Logically I know that the likelihood is that the scan will be normal: I didn't have metastases before, I didn't have nodes before and I have been on treatment. There is no rational reason why the scan should have anything on it, but I am worried that it will. You cannot fight emotion with reason — it just doesn't work.

FRIDAY 17 JANUARY

I have consistently said that I am afraid and that I hope that the fear would get better with every negative scan and scope that I have. Only the results weren't negative. There is a lesion on my liver. The radiologist and oncologist think it is low risk and is likely to be a fatty deposit, which is something which can occur in relation to the chemotherapy, but they can't be sure. Add to that my ongoing fever, which I have now had since the surgery, and I need to have another PET scan and an MRI.

All I really heard was "lesion on your liver". I know they said it is likely to be nothing but that is all I really heard. Again the battle between rational and emotional is waging: rational that it will be nothing, emotional that it will be everything. Yet again emotion is winning.

I desperately, desperately wanted a clean scan, a clean slate, for this to be over, but I am back in the land of uncertainty, waiting. I hate waiting, I hate not knowing the answer. It isn't what I hoped for.

It is now 4.20 a.m. Sleep is often the first thing to go.

SATURDAY 18 JANUARY

I ran away. Literally and physically. My husband came home from work, we got the kids and ran away to a hotel for the night. I have never run away before, in the way that we went yesterday, to get away from something. I haven't even run with regards to this cancer – I have stood up and faced it all head on. I was suddenly in a position where I had nothing to do but wait and worry, nothing to keep busy with.

We didn't have anything planned for today as I thought I would be recovering from the port being removed, which will now happen at some later date, I hope. Distraction was required, and a night in a hotel to top up my reserves and remember that we have a life outside of this was really helpful.

A swimming pool to keep the kids happy and a hotel breakfast – what more could you want?

SUNDAY 19 JANUARY

This week I will have a PET scan, an MRI scan and then will see the oncologist for the results. I am going to these appointments alone.

I appreciate that I have written here on various occasions, and indeed discussed often in therapy that I feel alone, that others cannot truly understand how I feel, or what my experience has been. Even with other cancer patients, we all will have had different experiences. I have been surrounded by family and friends, have been accompanied to everything I would let them come to, and yet I have felt alone.

I got into a bit of a routine though. I would travel to chemo myself and one of my parents would pick me up but I tended to see the oncologist alone. My husband and parents both asked over and over if I was sure I wanted to go alone today and tomorrow but I do. They said all the things I tell patients, that it is helpful to have a loved one if it is bad news, that other people will hear and remember differently to you, that I will forget and not be able to concentrate. I counter them all – I can ring you, I can write things down, I can email or ring with questions later. I want the opportunity to process whatever is coming my way, hopefully to feel the relief and joy, or not and to scream in my car instead. I need to deal with it myself, I need to have just a minute where it is all about me. I love my family, I really do, but they are all worried and frightened for me and I cannot help them with their emotions. I cannot feel the extra burden of their hopes and fears when I go to appointments. So I go alone.

Although I get almost unbearably anxious in the days leading up to an appointment, by the time I am sitting in the waiting room I am entirely calm. The doctor wall goes up; it is rather like scrubbing up to assist in an emergency C-section, or waiting for an ambulance to come screaming up to A & E. You know it is urgent, you know it could be extremely serious, or awful and distressing, or frightening. You know all of this and yet you are calm and in control and just keep going, systematically, allowing your training to take over – you just get on and do.

It is almost Pavlovian in a way – you are so drilled, for example, in doing life support that you do it almost automatically. You carry on, you plan, you are always thinking about next steps, but in the moment where everyone else panics and chaos could reign, your job is to be calm and in control. I use that wall, that skill, and go in feeling calm and ready. Tell me what you know, tell me what to do next.

TUESDAY 21 JANUARY

It isn't over till the fat lady sings and quite frankly she hasn't even left the changing room yet. Good news first – we always start with the good news, don't we? Sort of buoys you up for the bad news that might come next! There is no spread to the liver. There is some scarring and fibrosis on the liver and some fatty deposits but these will be due to the chemotherapy. Apparently it is very common after this kind of chemotherapy and due to the wonderful regenerative properties of the liver it will reverse and go back to normal.

Despite waiting for whatever was about to come next, some part of my brain was fascinated by this new medical knowledge; I didn't know that, how interesting! The rest of me was still listening to him talk, delivering the maybe-not-so-good news. The PET scan showed one lesion lighting up. The professor was talking and after a sentence or two I interrupted, asking him to repeat what he said to ensure I heard it right. I had twenty-seven nodes removed during the surgery and they were all negative so how do I have a node now? Well, I may or may not. Nodes become active for all kinds of reasons, including infection and inflammation – this doesn't necessarily mean cancer.

There was always going to be only one question I was going to ask next: but what if it does? The answer is that we don't know as yet and the guidance would be to repeat the scan in four–six weeks' time and then review. If it has stayed the same or grown then we will have to go and cut it out but it could just disappear again. I asked if I would need more chemo, and he swerved the question with "Let's wait and see". Does that mean yes?

There is good news here: there is no spread to the liver. But while that anxiety dissipates, it is replaced with the next about the nodes. Nodes are like the traffic lights of the immune system – once cancer has gone to a node, the lights turn to green and it can travel to the rest of your body. There is an urge to say "Just take it out" – in fact, I did say that – but it is a surgery and this could just be an incidental finding. I have to wait.

Did I mention I do not enjoy living in the land of uncertainty and waiting?

FRIDAY 24 JANUARY

Ben and I do not hide things from our children, or lie to them – generally kids know when something is up anyway! But I don't currently know what to tell them. The eldest two asked what the scans showed and I simply replied that I have to have more scans next month. I don't know what else to say. They don't need to carry this uncertainty and anxiety for the next month. They don't need to hold my fears, so it seems better to just tell them that we have to wait.

MONDAY 27 JANUARY

I had a procedure to remove my port today. Oddly enough, up until the scans last week this was something I was almost looking forward to. Not the discomfort, nor the grogginess from the sedation or feeling sore for a week or so, but it represented the end. The port coming out meant no more treatment – it was something that I viewed as positive. While that is still the case, it is tainted by the fact that I may need more treatment, that we might need to put it back, or use something else, that it isn't over yet.

As for the procedure, I am an old hand now, gown on backward, dressing gown on top, compression stockings, slipper socks on top. All jewellery off, glasses off, hair under a net and away we go! See you in an hour or so. It is odd in a way that time passes and you have no idea about it!

Bit sore now, as to be expected. I just wanted to feel relief and joy that it was out, and at the moment I can't.

WEDNESDAY 29 JANUARY

Oh joy… bowel prep day… again.

This will be the third occasion that I have done bowel prep and I will be doing it at least once a year forever and ever amen. Only I was a bit nervous about it as when I have done it before, I got diagnosed with cancer, or was about to have big surgery, and those times it really hurt – I mean it *hurt* and I was a nauseous, vomiting wreck, or a wretched, retching wretch!

This is less likely to happen this time as it was probably due to the cancer almost obstructing my bowel but I drank the prep with an element of trepidation. It definitely worked better this time; last time it took about five hours to start to work and this time we had lift-off after an hour!

We need to come up with a better way of emptying your entire colon than this! Today's prep involved drinking four pints of the disgusting stuff and rather a lot of time on the toilet. I mean a lot!!

THURSDAY 30 JANUARY

Pre-scope: It should be normal. I know rationally it should be normal, he cut it all out, but I can't sleep and I go over it over and over again in my head. The last and only other time I have had a scope they told me it was cancer and to be honest that was a pretty traumatic day. I am yet to have a normal scan, I am yet to be told I am in the all-clear, and heading back to a scope is worrying. I know he will tell me it will be OK, but everyone keeps telling me that the next scan or test will be normal and thus far they have all been wrong. I will be devastated if it is back already.

Post-scope: A clean scope, no evidence of cancer. I thought I would feel elated but all I feel is exhausted. This was supposed to be the last thing that I had to go through; if it was clear we would be done. But the PET scan and positive node mean that it isn't, and now I need to wait another month to hear if it has gone and what we do next. So the scope felt like just another hurdle to get over but not the end. It is relentless and the last two weeks have been draining. When will I be done, when can I ring the bell, when will it be over?

"Ringing the bell" signifies that you have finished your treatment, that you are in remission, or cancer-free. In some hospitals and clinics there is an actual bell and when someone rings it everyone claps and cheers. There has been some opposition to the bell, from cancer patients undergoing treatment, whose best hope is to live with their cancer, not to recover from it or reach remission, that it is difficult for them to hear others ring the bell. I understand this: from their point of view it seems hugely insensitive. There isn't a bell where I have treatment, but there is a metaphorical bell in my head, a bell I desperately, desperately want to ring, to cheer for myself.

SATURDAY 1 FEBRUARY

Today is my husband's fortieth birthday and tonight we are having a joint fortieth birthday party, admittedly belatedly for me. Fifty friends and family, cocktails and dancing – what more do you need? Below is my speech:

Today is Ben's birthday. Happy birthday, Ben. His fortieth and belatedly mine and we wanted to celebrate. A celebration of this kind in Ben's family usually ends up with someone singing or performing musically in some way; be warned that I won't be doing that, but am pretty sure I will end up crying, though many of you have all seen that anyway!

I also wanted to have this party to say thank you, to all of you, family and friends who make up the community and world we live in. For all your help and support over the past nine months, which have not been particularly fun! For all those kindnesses given without asking, for everyone who took the kids on play dates, who walked them to school, who bought bread, flowers and more. For everyone who offered a meal rota (and there were four of you within ten minutes of me sending a text about my cancer), though many of you were horrified that I wouldn't be able to eat for about a week – it is the Jewish mother in us all! For all of you who offered and offered, over and over again, even when I said no repeatedly, so I knew that you were still there, waiting to help. For all the touches on my shoulder in the playground that said you were there, caring and showing it. For the multitude of small kindnesses that made more difference than you will ever know, I want to thank you all.

Now, as many of you know, my husband can be a bit of a curmudgeon and would prefer to stay at home on a Saturday night than attend any party, probably including his own! He would often say when we were invited to a fortieth, fiftieth, ninetieth, "Why are we going? It is just a celebration of the fact that whoever it was hasn't died yet – how is that worth recognizing, just not dying?" Well, the truth is that some of us have to work harder than others at not dying. I would love to be able to tell you that I am completely cancer-free and that that period in our lives is over, but currently it is not and there is a bit of a way to go until we are out of the woods. But tonight is about Ben and his birthday, and also a recognition of the fact that no one died, that I am surviving. I can't think of anything more worth celebrating.

WEDNESDAY 5 FEBRUARY

I wanted to end this diary with my party on Saturday night, cancer-free and ready to start the next phase of my life. Instead I am waiting. Yet whatever happens at my scan in March, whatever is coming next, I have this month to be me and get on, keep moving forward. And so I do, but all the while, I wait.

JUNE 2020

I have often wondered how cancer patients ever got used to the sword of Damocles hanging over their heads. Will it come back? Am I safe? I wondered how I would come to terms with living with that same worry. I had hoped that in time, as I got further and further away from treatment with more and more negative scans, it would get easier to deal with.

Unfortunately I am not yet in that position. The node or mass they have been observing has continued to grow, albeit slowly. I have had various scans, biopsies and more, and the answers are inconclusive. It is a dilemma: the instinct of the oncologists is to take it out, in case it is cancer; the instinct of the surgeons is that it would be a huge surgery, even bigger than before, and not to subject me to that, in case it is not cancer. No one has the answer to the one question I ask: do I have cancer or not?

Specialist and even more specialist opinions are sought by the doctors, as this is an unusual dilemma. They all agree that the psychological burden of continued uncertainty is significant and should not be underestimated. Add into this a global coronavirus pandemic, the likes of which we have not seen in our lifetimes, and I think anyone with cancer feels that they are between a rock and a hard place. To continue with treatment is risky; to not continue is risky. I do not have to shield – I am not in active treatment – but was advised to be more cautious.

The surgeons recommended a laparoscopy, keyhole surgery – not to reach the mass, which they would not be able to do via keyhole, but to check if there is additional spread not seen on the scans. If there isn't, we have more time, to wait and scan again in the summer and operate if it grew further in the autumn. Major surgery which would require an ICU stay in combination with a global pandemic is to be avoided if possible! So in May this year I had further surgery, keyhole surgery with a hospital stay, and that is where you really feel the impact of the pandemic. I have written here about feeling alone with cancer, that no matter how many people I surround myself with I am essentially doing this alone. Only now, I really was: there's no one to sit with you while you wait for surgery, no one to hold your hand or stroke your hair when you come round. The nurses were kind, so, so kind, and I am incredibly grateful for their care, but being alone adds another layer of cruelty to the situation. Despite this, I am fortunate that my cancer was diagnosed pre lockdown, when so many people will have delayed diagnoses due to the pandemic, and that I had surgery during the crisis, when others have had treatment or trials delayed or stopped.

I returned home to three children off school, lockdown and recovery. It seems even harsher that my kids are getting used to the uncertainty about the cancer, to it not being over as well as to a new world where they don't go to school or see family or friends. I have tried to protect them from the minutiae – for example, they haven't accompanied me to appointments. Only in lockdown we can't leave the younger two at home so when my husband drove me to surgery or pre-op appointments they came too. We had a lovely time, singing at the tops of our lungs in the car, laughing, being together. It made the contrast of being alone in hospital even more stark.

The surgery did not show further spread. Again, we wait, this time with the potential of a big, scarier surgery up ahead, which would probably require a temporary stoma and, if cancerous, another round of chemo. I wanted to ring the bell, metaphorical or not, to declare to one and all that my cancer was gone and my treatment was finished. But maybe for me there won't be a decisive moment. I am afraid, really afraid; I don't think that before I had the opportunity to be, or the true experiential knowledge of what this may involve, and now I really do. The fear is becoming all-encompassing, yet I wait, and find a way to live during the wait.

There is some certainty: if it grows, I will have the surgery and end up with no cancer, and if this mass wasn't cancerous then I still end up with no cancer, just more surgeries. But there is a greater certainty: I can survive this. I will survive this. My body is strong, perhaps stronger than my mind; it heals, it gets fit, it persists. So do I – I have to continue, keep going, moving forward.

AUGUST 2020

As the next set of scans approached I was aware of my anxiety levels getting higher, peaking not at the time of the scans themselves but when waiting for the results.

The lesion has grown. Not a lot, but it is growing and needs to be removed. The surgical teams had their multidisciplinary team meetings to discuss the best approach to reach the lesion. The urologists wondered if they could get to it from the back, the radiologists by imaging guided biopsy, but in the end as the lesion is close to the small bowel the colorectal surgeons won the toss as to who would be the lucky ones to cut me open, again!

This surgery is big, really big. It's known as a laparotomy, which involves cutting open your whole abdomen, in a line from under your breastbone to above your pubic region. They may have to remove some small bowel but hopefully they'll be able to leave the large intestine where the previous cancer was alone. This means that my risk of needing a stoma is small. They will remove various bits and pieces in there including part of my abdominal wall muscles as the lesion seems to be invading into them. I will also get a form of chemotherapy called HIPEC (hyperthermic intraperitoneal chemotherapy) where they will put some chemotherapy directly into my tummy before sewing me back up. However, it isn't all bad; they have decided to leave my ovaries in – every cloud has a silver lining!

I'm gonna say it again, this is big. A few nights in intensive care and probably around two weeks in hospital. There was talk of various different lines, bowel prep, bowel rest and far more. It is a lot to absorb, to take in, and if I knew that last time the surgery was big and bad, this is bigger and badder. I truly know now what there is to be afraid of.

I have been waiting for a long time, living with uncertainty of what the lesion is and what the plan will be. The waiting has been exhausting. Now we have a plan, and however daunting it may be there is an element of peace and acceptance with it, at least a decision has been made. It is time to bring it on.

Now I wait for a bed…

THURSDAY 3 SEPTEMBER

Today I took my children as an "end of holidays and home school" treat to a high ropes course where you are attached by a harness and progress through various obstacles. The littlest is now five and, like many small children, constantly narrates her life to herself. She lives in her own operetta singing away to herself about her day. We approached an enormous net, about 20 feet in the air, which you had to scramble across. She looked at it and said out loud, but very clearly to herself and not to me, "ooh, that's a big net" and without hesitation, without even glancing back at me, put her foot on to the net and took a step. As she went across I could hear her: "one step, just one step", "one step, nearly there", "one step".

Out of the mouths of babes… I need to do the same: "one step, just one step."

FRIDAY 11 SEPTEMBER

The date is set for a week's time. I have to stay at home and self-isolate before surgery in order to decrease the chances of contracting coronavirus pre-operatively. I will also have to have swabs 48 hours before at the pre-operative assessment clinic. One of my coping mechanisms is to keep busy, to keep going and distract myself with work and family and life, staying at home, even though we have all been doing just that for months due to coronavirus. There is too much time to think, it's hard on the head.

The coronavirus pandemic has made everything more complicated and the costs of Covid-19 will be seen for many years to come. There is the health cost related to the virus itself, to other conditions where treatment was delayed due to the pandemic, all the way to the physical and mental health effects of a recession. The psychological burden of the pandemic, on all of us, is not to be underestimated. Whether we live alone or with family, were furloughed, kept working or were made redundant, there has been a mental health burden. One of the places that this is felt most acutely is in hospital when as a patient you are not allowed visitors. Indeed, being afraid of being alone was one of the reasons I delayed having this larger surgery back in May.

Yet here we are, months on, in exactly the same position. The virus has not gone away and now I am heading for about two weeks in hospital with another ICU stay and I will be doing so alone. If I am lucky my husband will be allowed in for an hour or so a week. My children will not be able to come and see me, to see with their own eyes to prove to themselves that I am OK. Two weeks is an awfully long time in the mind of a child. My husband, parents and siblings will not be able to comfort me and I feel this loss more than any fear of surgery. I accept that I need surgery, that this is going ahead, that the recovery will be tough and long but I am afraid to do it alone. The response to that is that I won't be alone, that there will be doctors and nurses, but we all know that it is not the same.

Technology helps. I hope to still read at bedtime to my children, be at the family dinner table over video call. I can receive messages all day from people if I need and want to, but I remember finding that difficult initially last time. Phoning someone seems to require that you have something to say. When Ben or my parents sat in the room, they could hold my hand and say absolutely nothing at all and it was enough.

I brace myself. I try to prepare mentally. I try to remember all the things that helped or didn't help last time, even though it still hurts to remember. I breathe. Yet the fear is still there.

WEDNESDAY 16 SEPTEMBER

Today I went on television to talk about my cancer. I appreciate that this sounds almost bizarre – most people don't do that! It raised the question of why, why do I now need to tell after spending so long keeping it private, not a secret, but private.

The answer is complex, but I need to do something positive as a result of what has happened to me. Perhaps, in some small way, I can help someone out there feel less alone. That by showing my own vulnerability I can help others see or accept their own, or recognize that their loved ones may be feeling a similar way. I don't speak for all patients, that would be extraordinarily arrogant, but my experience as a patient and as a doctor who cares for patients is that many of us go through the same gamut of emotions.

Transference is the term used to describe the situation when you pick up on someone else's emotions and begin to feel that way yourself. For example, when someone is sad and you feel sad too, you feel a tiny fraction of their sadness in yourself. This means that when you express your fears, your sadness or your anger about a situation to your loved ones, they feel a tiny fragment of that too. And it makes them uncomfortable, it hurts them and consciously or not they want to fix it, to make it better, to make you better, because they desperately want you not to feel it too. This is when you get the messages of positivity, of reassurance, of support. As a patient you are told that you are strong, that you are brave, that you will be fine.

I know all of this… yet I am also scared.

You can be brave and scared, resolute and frightened, strong and vulnerable, angry and accepting all at the same time. Personally, and we all are different, right now I don't need to be told that I will be OK, that I have the strength to do this: I know these things, but what I need is to be heard. I need you to hear that I am afraid and to sit with me in the fear for just a little bit. You can't make this experience better for me, so instead come and join me in it, help me feel less alone.

After the interview there was a sense of peace, that nothing was hidden anymore. Not that it was a secret, but it was private and I needed to be ready to share. It has taken a long time to accept that this is part of my story, but it is, and now I can use that to hopefully help others.

THURSDAY 17 SEPTEMBER

The last supper… again! Tomorrow I will take the bowel prep and start the process.

Surgery is the first step to recovery here; it hurts in order to heal.

WEDNESDAY 30 SEPTEMBER

Hello from the other side! It has been a while. Today is day eleven post-op and the first time I have felt well enough to write.

For the first time, I think I signed a consent form that included risk of death. That risk is always there, no matter what you are doing, but I don't remember seeing it written so starkly on a consent form before. Perhaps I blocked it out from my memory, but there it was: 1 in 100 chance of dying. You sign anyway and hope you are not signing your life away but rather signing on for a new one.

I awoke in recovery, thankfully not remembering the point where they removed the breathing tube, and in between vomiting, I asked the same questions I asked before. Did you get it? Yes. Do I have a bag? No. Relief.

There then followed ten days and nine nights in the intensive care unit. An incredibly long and tough period of time which I am yet to truly process in my head – this too will take time, lots of talking, writing and therapy!

Ten days, nine nights. I haven't been away on holiday for longer than that time since our honeymoon fifteen years ago. A couple of days ago on a video call with my parents I asked them what they had done the previous week. My father responded that they had kept themselves busy and waited for the time to pass until I came back to them. I have done the same: waited, waited and persisted and waited until I have come back. The world outside trundled on, with the coronavirus pandemic continuing, while I remained in my own personal little lockdown in ICU.

The dreaded first night post-operatively was indeed awful but over the following two or three days I was unable to keep my eyes open for more than about ten minutes at a time. Like a newborn baby I would simply drift off to sleep, although I felt like I was fighting to be awake, and needed to be reassured that it was OK to need so much rest and sleep. This was likely to be the effect of the chemotherapy and although I was warned it would be like being run over by a steamroller I think I underestimated the level of exhaustion which would follow. Even now looking back I can see how little I messaged on my phone, how I video called the children for about a minute at most. I was incapable of doing more.

The ICU staff were phenomenal and worked extremely hard to ensure that the problems of my previous admission did not arise, but despite having one-to-one nursing care I have never felt so lonely in my entire life. Not alone but lonely. The lack of visitors has an enormous impact on your psychological well-being. Yes, there is technology, which helps certainly but it requires energy to talk, something to say and the ability to take a big enough breath to throw your voice slightly when on speakerphone.

For the first week I saw my children at most for a minute twice a day to say "have a good day at school" and "I love you, good night". I could not manage more. What did cut through the loneliness though were letters. I had asked my friends and family to write to me and every day the post arrived at about four o'clock, like a lifeline of connection to the outside world, to my life. It doesn't matter what they wrote (and what they wrote is to be kept and treasured indefinitely), it is that they took the time to write, and write reams, or choose a particular picture or quote to send to me. This takes more time than a text, or finding a meme; it takes care, it takes love. And I felt that love, through the ICU, through the illness, recovery, global pandemic and all. Letters to make you laugh, to make you cry (though both physically hurt in equal measure!), letters that you can cherish and read over and over and feel for just that short period of time less alone. If letter-writing is a dying art, I propose a revival!

Ben was allowed into the ICU for one visit, in full personal protective equipment, mainly to protect me from him, and I have never been so glad to see anyone in my entire life. You know those pictures of elderly couples sitting on benches by the sea, holding hands and looking content? The ones where you think "sweet" and hope to be like that some day? We sat and held hands, his gloved, mine still clutching the blessed pain-relief clicker of the patient-controlled analgesia and I felt safe and at peace.

◆

We mark the passage of time in various ways, with birthdays and festivals, with each year, or the start of the new school year, with weekends and parties and more. On a more day-to-day level we mark time passing by seeing the light of day, not necessarily always a sunny sky in England but natural daylight to be followed by the darkness of night. We break up the day with work, or school or play, with mealtimes and at the most basic level by responding to the needs of our own bodies: for food, to go to the toilet! In ICU for me, every single one of these markers was removed: no daylight, no night-time quiet, no food, not even the urge to go to the loo due to the catheter and a completely silent, resting, healing bowel. The only marker of change was the 12-hourly nursing shift change, and to be honest there was no real difference between 8 a.m. and 8 p.m. where that was concerned. You are aware it is night and try to sleep more but the sleep is fractionated by noise, and pain and being attended to. You doze in the day, you try to find items to track the passage of time that are more than your watch, though you use that to know when to ring home before school, or to await the post.

Put simply, you wait. You wait for your astounding, resilient body to begin to heal. Sure it needs help, an awful lot of help, but essentially you wait and waiting is hard. During my last big operation I was warned of excruciating agony before the first time you pass wind, which I did not experience. This time, with my intestines entirely asleep for over a week, the pain as they began to wake up was unimaginable. There were various separate pains – pains from the drains when they pulled, pains from the large cut down your middle, aches from being hunched over and more – but these were internal intestinal pains, cramping waves of agony that would come and go for a few minutes at a time followed by an awareness of air in the gut, like your tummy rumbling, but it took a few days before the gas passed. When the pain came, nothing helped at all: not the epidural, not the patient-controlled analgesia, nothing.

Your world dissolves into the molten ball of lava in your tummy and still you wait, you wait for it to pass.

I often use time both as a patient and as a doctor, and although it is difficult to wait, time heals a great deal. When time seems too indefinite we shrink it – just get through today, or until home time – and sometimes we need to decrease that even further – get through the next hour, or even the next five minutes. We plan the rewards for getting through: nice food, a hot bath, rubbish TV or a good book; we distract ourselves from our pains be they physical or psychological and in doing so time passes. In those moments, in that pain, even 5 minutes was too large a space of time; I could not even count to 60 for one minute or even to ten. I was down to counting every single breath. And telling myself to take the next one. And the next. Single breaths that needed the voice in my head to say *keep going, just one more, it will pass*: one breath, one step, one step. With my children as markers at the beginning and end of each day, I would take one breath at a time until I reached them. One breath, and then another. I hope to never be in that position again.

THURSDAY 1 OCTOBER

There are important medical skills, difficult to define and to teach, that are born of experience. If you ask doctors what the most important part of the patient examination is most of them will say "eyeballing the patient", sometimes called the "end of the bed-o-gram". Put simply this is when you look at a patient and know that something is wrong, even if you are not sure exactly what it is yet.

This feeling, this awareness, is clinical intuition and is often due to experience, but we have it for ourselves and for our children, an awareness that something isn't right. For the first few days the ICU doctors would ask me how I was and when I replied they would agree that I did indeed look terrible! What that terrible is is hard to explain, more than pallor, sometimes a greyish or greenish tinge to the skin, sometimes the obvious effort it takes for someone to speak. There was a period of time on the first night when my blood pressure kept falling and while it was being treated the doctor who was issuing instructions stood and watched. It was when he pronounced that I looked better that I knew things were stabilizing. Now when the doctors walk in they look at me and say that I look well. Sure, pale and tired, but well.

As I progressed my ability to stay awake for slightly longer periods of time, to mobilize better, to concentrate, all improved. Most importantly for me my ability to engage with my children came back. It was only after I was out of the ICU that the phone could be propped up on the kitchen table and I was able to ask questions I would normally ask during dinner time: who did what at school, who they played with, what the best part of their days were, with them wanting to show me their work and talk to me. I was able to listen to piano practice and even play a quiz game. This more than anything tells me I am getting better.

When I awoke from surgery I had a nasogastric tube, a catheter, two surgical drains, a central line, other drips, monitors and more. After a week in ICU these started to be removed, first one drain, then the central line, then more, and the more that are removed, the better you must be as you don't need them any more! In a way each of these removals is a little hurdle that must be jumped, to be endured, as they can be painful or make you anxious, but they are to be celebrated as wins. The biggest victory of all was the removal of the nasogastric tube (or NG tube – which runs from your nose to your stomach to drain your stomach contents). This tube is essential, but it is not a comfortable thing to live with, though I am assured that people do get used to it in time, or that the thinner more flexible kind which is used to feed people is easier to tolerate. I could always feel it move when I swallowed, it irritated my throat, it made my nausea immeasurably worse. I was aware of it constantly, perhaps even in my sleep as the one time I was given a sleeping pill I must have slept deeper and woke up with the securing tape wrapped around my hand and the tube, which I could still feel in my throat, clenched within it. I barely dared to move as I alerted the nurse. Thankfully I had only pulled it out about 10 centimetres (it was inserted approximately 60 centimetres deep) but I had to sit up and swallow water as they pushed it further in through my nose back into my stomach, which was painful and nauseating and horrible. Yet you tolerate it, you tolerate it all, because that is how you get better. When the NG tube was finally taken out, eight long days after surgery, apparently I was beaming even as my head came up to look at the nurse. Instant relief.

A couple of days ago I started to eat again and today the parenteral nutrition, the broken-down components of food which are infused continuously into my veins, has been stopped. The nurses remove the last line, the PICC line, and that is it; I am no longer attached to a drip stand and fluids, I can get dressed without having to be detached and reattached, or the drips passed through sleeves or my bra. I can walk without having to push the heavy stand along with me, I can get out of bed (or rather heave myself out) to go to the toilet without having to unplug machines and then plug them back in. Free from lines and attachments, my systems are go, my body can stand alone.

A free woman indeed, free in many, many ways because for the first time in the past sixteen months I am able to say, with complete confidence, that I am cancer free. I do not have cancer any more.

The results came back and showed that the lesions the surgeons removed were not malignant spread but abscesses, which are a pocket of infection. These abscesses had a hard wall around them which explains why I have not been unwell this whole time as the infection was kept in one place, but may also have been contributing to my temperature.

My initial response to this news was twofold: a combination of relief and feeling completely overwhelmed by this most enormous undertaking. On the scans it looked like cancer, they were growing and spreading and invading, and it acted like cancer; there was no choice, it had to be removed. Hindsight is 20/20, so perhaps the internal chemotherapy could have been avoided, but we took the most appropriate course of action at the time. I know this, I know we had no choice, I know we waited and waited to do this surgery, until we could not wait any more.

A week after hearing this news my feelings are firmly in the relief zone. The surgery had to be undertaken and the results are as good as they could have been, not malignant, not cancer. My prognosis returns to be as good as it was when there was no spread to the nodes, 90–95 per cent survival at five years. A large undertaking yes, a big surgery, but from now, from right now, the only way forward is recovery.

This is it. This is me ringing that metaphorical bell. I have survived, I will survive.

My name is Philippa, I am 40 years old and I no longer have cancer.

I am cancer-free.

Even as I write that I know that I am not entirely free, that there will be scans and follow-ups, with anxiety and concerns ongoing. Others will never be able to write that sentence and for that I am sorry; we must do more, we must learn more about this disease, we must raise awareness and continue to find new treatments. The majority of us though will recover fully and I am now incredibly grateful to now be able to count myself as in that group.

I no longer have cancer.

I am cancer-free.

It feels good.

AFTERWORD

In the end one has to think, do you feel lucky?

Is it lucky to have colon cancer (or indeed any cancer) at the age of thirty-nine? Almost certainly not. Is it lucky to have something, whether or not they have got it all, which affected my quality of life, and will potentially shorten my life, even if not by much? Definitely not. Is it lucky to have to have six-monthly scans and annual colonoscopies? Nope.

But is it lucky to have colon cancer (or indeed any cancer) at the age of thirty-nine? Perhaps also yes. I am young, I am healthy, my heart and my body are fit and well, apart from the frigging cancer of course, and so I will heal far quicker than someone older with other illnesses or conditions. I bounced back far quicker than an eighty-year-old. I got back to physical fitness, though I will inevitably be changed psychologically.

I am lucky it was found. For this I am grateful, hugely and overwhelmingly grateful. I emailed the gynaecologist from hospital to tell him, for I believe that it is due to his skill that this was picked up so early.

I went for pelvic pain and had multiple reasons why this could be, most likely related to adhesions from previous surgery. The vascular glue used to stop the bleeding after the C-section from my littlest had essentially stuck me together with scar tissue. These adhesions did not show on either ultrasound or MRI scan, neither of which are great at showing them but still.

Perhaps another surgeon would have gone for a laparoscopy and then seen the adhesions, of which there were lots, all divided during my surgery, and said job done. I could have been a chronic pelvic pain patient, with no known cause for my pain. He so, so easily could have been reassured by the adhesions in a way, and would never ever think to look in the bowel.

I would have presented eventually as my cancer was already partially obstructing my bowel but it would have likely presented in acute bowel obstruction, which is a surgical emergency, and doing anything as an emergency has poorer outcomes than electively. By that point the cancer would have been far bigger and may well have spread.

So I am lucky, lucky to have had a clever gynaecologist who thought to tick all the boxes, who thought to check my bowel, lucky to have a colorectal surgeon who found it and removed it. The oncologist said it was a hugely lucky find, that in the vast majority of cases, without obvious symptoms and with symptoms which could so easily be attributed to something else, it could so easily have been missed.

That the cancer was discovered? Lucky. Oh so lucky. And it was picked up just before I went into complete obstruction, which is a surgical emergency – hugely fortunate.

That I needed a major surgery? Unlucky. But that I had a cancer found at a point where complete surgical removal was possible? Lucky.

No metastases? Oh, so gratefully lucky.

No nodes? Hugely lucky.

No ileostomy bag? Temporary or not... lucky.

In medicine everything is a balance, and as doctors we put every choice we make on the scale – risks vs benefits, pros vs cons, the number needed to treat vs the number needed to cause harm. When I take a blood sample you could bleed out if you have no platelets, when you take a medication you could go into anaphylactic shock – every decision is a weighing up of the balances. For me, in this scenario, was I lucky to have colon cancer at age thirty-nine? Probably yes. Far luckier than having this same cancer found at forty-one, forty-three or even later. This is the mindset I choose to take, one of gratitude and luck over the despair I felt at the beginning. For I am lucky, so fortunate, in so many ways.

APPENDICES

THE JUST-IN-CASE-LETTER

The first "just in case" letter, written 11 May 2019

11ᵗʰ May 2019

To my world Harrison, Edward & Madeline,

How do I start? How do I write a lifetime of love in a letter? As this is a just in case letter I am not going to try but just in case the operation doesn't go as planned I wanted to write this letter.

I love you.

I loved you from before you were born, when you were two lines on a pregnancy test. I loved being pregnant with you, when it was just you and me together and I loved you the moment you arrived. No matter what happens to you in your lives remember this, I have always loved you and I will always love you, whether I am here or not my love will not go away.

Harrison, Edward and Madeline you are the most important things in my life. You have given me purpose, a reason for being and the reason for striving to be the best I can be. I am only sorry that I have failed you if I am no longer here and for any pain this brings you. But I haven't really gone, like it or not I am inside all of you, you can hear my voice in your head, you know what I am going to say!

You are all amazing children and will be astounding adults in your own way, whatever that may be. Look after each other, there is nothing more important than family, always be there for each other, always.

Be happy, be kind, be brave, be whomever and whatever you wish, be happy, be healthy, be safe.

Listen to Daddy and to all the people who love you, and there are lots. You are lucky to have so many people who love you.

I have absolute faith that you will be fine, that you will thrive and flourish. I haven't really gone, I am in your heart, your mind, your soul.

Know that I love you, that you are adored and loved,
        Mummy

OP PACKING TIPS
(THE NON-MATERNITY EDIT)

There are lots of guides as to what to pack in your hospital bag when you are having a baby – what is for you, what is for your partner, what is for baby – but a lack of information about what to take when planning a major op. A few home comforts can make all the difference. This is my suggested prep list to pack for the worst holiday ever:

- Technology – whichever devices you use to stay in touch, watch TV, etc. Chargers and charger packs.
- Download audiobooks, podcasts or music as you may not be well enough to concentrate on reading a book but may be able to manage an audio version. Don't forget headphones.
- Magazines, books, adult colouring books, etc. in case you do feel up to it.
- Top up your phone data if the hospital WiFi isn't any good.
- A small amount of money – not so much you worry about it being taken, but enough for hospital TV, etc., which can be surprisingly expensive.
- Any medication you take.
- Flip-flops for the shower.
- Dressing gown, slippers, changes of nightwear – even wearing day PJs and night ones can make you feel better!
- If you are having abdominal surgery then bring on the Bridget Jones pants! You may need bigger knickers – size

up and full briefs, not bikinis, so the edges don't irritate the wounds.

- Soft bras, as you may be swollen in comparison to normal, to avoid the bras or wires digging in.
- Toiletries, including dry shampoo and baby wipes if you are too pooped for a shower, lip balm for dry lips, cream as your skin often gets dry, mints or other sweets for dry mouth – mint or lemon also often helps with nausea.
- Soft hairband to hold your hair off your face – even think about soft hair bobbles, basically nothing to irritate.
- Handheld fan – it is always so hot!
- If you are having abdominal surgery, take a small hand towel and roll it up very tightly and secure it with tape. Then, after the surgery, if you need or want to cough or sneeze, squeeze the rolled-up towel against your wound as hard as you can. You can't push hard enough to cause yourself any damage and the support it gives the wound means that coughing or sneezing hurts less.
- Something to uplift you – a photo of your kids, a favourite view or a quote.
- Set up a group WhatsApp or other chat so either one family member (or yourself if you are able) can update everyone in one go, otherwise you or they will spend their whole time on the phone.

HOME POST-OP TIPS

- Plan ahead. Make sure that you have plenty of paracetamol and/or ibuprofen (if allowed). Ensure that you have enough of your normal medications. You will be given medications to take home but you may need further painkillers, etc. and although your GP will be able to prescribe these you don't want to be caught short on a Friday night before a bank holiday weekend.

- Take the contact details of the ward, consultant's secretary, out-of-hours GP number, or just 111, your GP surgery's contact number, etc. and put them in an easily accessible place.

- Arrange supermarket home deliveries for a few weeks. You can always change the order but knowing you aren't going to run out of essentials (and treats!) is a blessing!

- If you are having bowel surgery then get in some nappy cream; if you are going more than normal you may get a sore bum!

- As a woman I often have a treatment for thrush in the bathroom cupboard, just in case; if you have lots of antibiotics as part of your treatment you may well get thrush, and again it can be useful knowing that a pessary/tablet/cream is there and you don't have to go and get one.

- Get some post-op clothes, maybe a size up, maybe loose baggy trousers and tops, especially if you have had abdominal surgery.

- Keep planning if that helps you. I may not have had the headspace for myself, for my friends, for visiting, etc. – all the headspace that I did have was for my kids. Arranging lifts when I couldn't drive, working out what my husband could do which fitted in with work, trying to work out when I might manage the twenty-minute walk to school (even if I get a lift back home), etc. If you can do so before the op, cooking and freezing meals is also useful – pulling out a frozen Bolognese and reheating it while cooking pasta still makes me feel like I am giving my kids home-cooked food (because I am!) but is easier than starting from scratch.

- If you know you are going to need a special diet after you are home then order it in. I didn't realize I would be eating ice cream and had to send someone to get it!

- Put in rest time. Consider a *Don't disturb* sign on the door saying, *Please don't ring between 1–3 p.m.* (as if your baby is asleep but you are the baby) and make sure you go to bed, even if it is to rest, not sleep.

- For rest times, or for times with kids when you are trying to be present, turn your phone on silent. Put an out of office on your email.

- Hospital beds are very versatile things and the electronic lift for your head or legs section is really useful. Put pillowcases on a few pillows to prop yourself up when at home and if you have had abdominal surgery don't forget to turn on your side and walk your legs off the bed before pushing yourself up – it is easier on the tummy muscles.

- Realize that if you stand at the side of the bed, slip off those loose, soft-waisted baggy trousers before sitting down, leaning to the side and lifting your legs up to lie down and have a nap, that when you roll back on to your side, walk your legs off the bed and heave yourself up again, that your feet will automatically be in the holes for your trousers for you to yank them back up. Feel inordinately pleased about this. In fact, this should be a life goal for many people.

- Keep walking – start little and often, slow and steady. Plan this into your day along with your rests.

- Try (and fail) to not get frustrated with yourself or push yourself too hard – you will get there.

GLOSSARY

Adhesion – when areas of internal scar tissue stick together, which can cause organs to become stuck to the scar tissue and stuck together.

Anastomosis – a join; for example, if you remove a section of bowel and sew the two ends of healthy bowel back together, the join is termed the anastomosis.

Benign – a growth which is not malignant, unlikely to be harmful.

Biopsy – when a sample of tissue is removed from a lesion (often with a needle) in order that the sample can be examined under a microscope to see what the lesion is made of, and whether or not it is malignant.

Bowel preparation – also called bowel prep – the medications taken to empty the large intestine before a colonoscopy or surgery.

BRCA genes – BReast CAncer genes 1 and 2 – associated with a higher risk of developing breast and other cancers, including ovarian cancer.

Chemotherapy – medication which is toxic to cancer cells.

Colectomy – a partial colectomy removes part of the colon; a pan or total colectomy removes the entire colon.

Colon – the large intestine.

Colonoscopy – a procedure in which a camera is inserted through the anus into the colon in order to visualize the colon itself; also shortened to scope.

CT scan – a computed tomography scan – involves X-rays to create an image of your organs (see Guide to Imaging Investigations).

Endoscopy – a medical procedure which involves a camera being inserted into the body in order to see inside. The shorthand term for endoscopy is a scope – see *colonoscopy*.

Histology – the study of looking at cells under the microscope to determine if they are malignant or benign.

Hyperthermic intraperitoneal chemotherapy (HIPEC) – a form of heated chemotherapy that is placed into the abdomen during surgery, which is used to treat cancer which has spread in the abdomen.

Laparoscopy – keyhole surgery – here small incisions are made into the abdomen, and a camera and other instruments are inserted to perform the surgery. Smaller cuts generally mean a quicker recovery than with traditional surgery.

Laparotomy – an open surgery on the abdomen, with one large incision. Due to the size of the incision, this generally has a longer recovery time than keyhole surgery.

Lesion – an area of abnormality in the body, this can be due to cancer or other disease or injury.

Lines – tubes placed into a vein or artery to take samples and deliver medications and fluids:

- **Arterial line** – a line into an artery, often the radial artery at the wrist; gives accurate readings of the gases in the blood.
- **Cannula** – a tube inserted into a vein through which medication is given; sometimes called a drip.
- **Central line** – a line into the big veins in the neck which goes all the way inside or just near the heart.
- **PICC line** – a long-lasting line or tube into a vein in the body. Ordinarily a cannula has to be changed every seventy-two hours to decrease risk of infection; a PICC line can stay for up to six months.

Lymph nodes – part of the lymphatic and immune systems in the body. Essentially the traffic lights of the body. If a cancer has not spread to the nodes then the traffic lights are red, the cancer cannot spread to other parts of the body; if the cancer has spread to the nodes, then the lights turn to green and the cancer can spread further.

Malignant – a growth which is cancerous.

Metastasis/metastases (singular/plural) – when a cancer has spread from the original site in the body to another area or other areas in the body.

MRI scan – magnetic resonance imaging scan – uses a large magnet to create an image of your organs (see Guide to Imaging Investigations).

Nasogastric tube (NG tube) – a tube from your nose which travels down the back of the throat, down the oesophagus into the stomach. This can be used to drain stomach contents, as in the case of intestinal obstruction, which may be caused by the temporary paralysis of the intestines post-surgery and is used on a temporary basis. Alternatively a thinner, more flexible tube can be used for longer periods of time in order to feed patients whose intestines are working but who may not be able to eat or swallow for another reason.

Nodes – see *lymph nodes*.

Patient-controlled analgesia (PCA) – a form of pain relief where the patient presses a button to release pain medication as and when they require it.

PET scan – positron emission tomography scan – uses a radioactive substance to visualize areas of unusual increased cellular activity in the body (see Guide to Imaging Investigations).

Polyp – a growth in the body; with regards to polyps in the colon, these initially are benign but over time may become malignant.

Port – see *portacath*.

Portacath – a medical device placed under the skin of the chest which is attached to a tube within a large vein; medications such as chemotherapy can be given via the port.

Cancer staging and grading – cancers are staged according to the size of tumour, if it has spread to the nodes and if there has been further spread (metastases). Grading refers to what the cancer cells look like when examined under a microscope – lower grade cancers tend to grow slower than higher grade cancers.

Stent – a tube inserted into a structure to keep it open. For example, a cardiac stent is inserted into a cardiac artery to keep it open. See also *ureteric stent*.

Stoma – an opening in the abdomen which is connected to the bowel or urinary system for waste (stool or urine) to be collected in a bag and removed from the body:
- **Colostomy** – the opening in the abdomen connects to the large intestine.
- **Ileostomy** – the opening in the abdomen connects higher up the digestive system to the small intestine. The waste

collected from an ileostomy is more liquid than that in a colostomy.

Suture – the medical term for a stitch, used to sew up incisions. Medical staples can also be used.

Total parenteral nutrition (TPN) – when you receive all the nutrients you require through your veins. Your intestines break down food into its component parts, such as lipids from fats. In TPN you are given the already broken-down nutrients directly into your vein, allowing your intestines to rest.

Tumour – a growth in the body which can be benign or malignant, often used by laypeople to mean cancer.

Ureteric stent – see *stent*, in this case to hold open and protect the ureter, the tube between the kidney and bladder.

THE PATIENT'S GUIDE TO IMAGING INVESTIGATIONS

I have now had a virtual smorgasbord of imaging. We as doctors often talk about imaging in terms of what it can show, or if it has risks like radiation, but what is it like to experience these tests?

- **X-ray** – the easiest of them all. No need to change into a hospital gown most of the time – just stand/sit/lie and an X-ray is taken. You feel absolutely nothing at all, bar the weight of the lead apron you may have to wear over your reproductive bits.
- **Ultrasound** – the next simplest, similar to what pregnant women have. You may or may not have to put on a gown. The worst bit of this is having the cold jelly spread on your belly or wherever. Sometimes they have to push a bit hard and if this is over your bladder you might feel like you need to wee. Can have a transvaginal scan, so inside the vagina; here a medical-type condom covers an ultrasound probe which is inserted into the vagina. It might feel a bit uncomfortable but isn't painful.
- **CT scan** – this one involves radiation (more than an X-ray), and you will need to change into a hospital gown. You lie on your back generally and your body is passed through what looks like a rather large doughnut. Your head is generally outside the machine, unless you are having a CT head scan, in which case your feet will be outside. Takes a few minutes. If having an abdominal or

chest CT, you may be given instructions about taking a breath in and holding your breath; the longest I had to do this for was eight seconds. Apart from following any breathing exercises, you stay as still as you can. The scan lasts up to about 10–15 minutes.

- **CT with contrast** – as for a CT above but a cannula is placed into your hand/arm and at some point an injection is given of contrast, which helps certain things show up on a scan. You may notice the following as the contrast is given, pretty immediately: a revolting metallic taste in your mouth, nausea, palpitations and, the most disconcerting of all, a feeling that you have wet yourself. You haven't but there can be a sensation of warmth spreading over your genitals as if you had. Even knowing this, I thought I had wet myself; the next time, even knowing that, I still found myself "squeezing" as if to stop myself wetting myself. It is pretty strange. Make sure you drink a lot afterwards to flush the contrast out of your system.

- **Ultrasound-guided or CT-guided biopsy** – this involves using either ultrasound or CT scans to see exactly where a lesion is and then using a needle to take a small biopsy. If it is ultrasound guided, you have the ultrasound as normal; if CT guided, you will have multiple CTs, so move in and out of the scanner during the procedure. The radiologist will talk to you the whole time, and it is important you stay still. They inject you with local anaesthetic first – this feels rather like a bee sting but then removes the pain of taking the biopsy, though you might feel some pressure as it is taken. After a few hours when the local anaesthetic wears off, you may have some discomfort where the biopsy was taken – using over-the-counter painkillers is fine (unless you have been told not to!).

- **MRI** – this one doesn't involve any radiation at all. It is essentially an enormous magnet in a tube. You will need to change into a hospital gown and remove all metal from your body, including earrings, watch, glasses, etc. If you have metal inside your body, such as a pacemaker, you can't have an MRI as the magnet is so strong it essentially would rip the pacemaker out of your body, which is not really ideal! So no metal at all, though my portacath in my chest was MRI safe. This time you lie down and may have a sort of cage placed over part of your body, for example your chest, which can feel quite restrictive. Then you are passed into the MRI machine, which is a tube. Now, I am small and am not claustrophobic and even I am aware that it is a small space, but in all the machines I have been in I have still been able to see the light on either end of the tube. MRI scans can take up to an hour so they often put music in headphones for you as the machine itself is rather loud and makes clunking noises and beeps. Again, for an abdominal MRI, you may be asked to hold your breath. I have had an MRI scan where I was told to exhale and hold my breath; in others it was the other way around, to inhale and hold my breath. You do your best and hold as long as you can.

- **MRI with contrast** – generally with something called gadolinium. Similar to the CT with contrast, this requires a drip in your hand or arm but tends to have no side effects at all – it just felt cold going in. Again, drink lots afterwards.

- **CT PET scan** – the largest amount of radiation of all of those discussed. Here you are injected with a radioactive tracer, which they deliver in a lead-lined box to stop the radiation leaking out, which always freaked me out a bit – protect everyone else with a lead-lined box but inject it into me! No side effects from the injection. You then lie in a darkened room for sixty to ninety minutes. I have had one where I wasn't allowed any stimulation at all and one where I was told I could still text/answer emails on my phone. The first radiographer said that stimulation from my phone would make my brain light up, and the second radiographer that my brain, heart, liver and kidneys always light up as they are always working! Either way, you sit or lie quietly and try not to move too much – if you do lunges, your quads will light up on the scan and they will think you have something there! You then go into a scanner which feels like a CT scan, but the difference between a CT PET scan and a CT scan is the injection of radiation so the images produced don't simply show the structure of your internal organs, but also areas of increased metabolic activity, generally areas which could represent infection or cancer.

Here's the thing: I have now had plenty of these scans and what I think is missing is something on the inside of the CT or MRI scanner. In only one machine I went in there was a complex art design, where you can see all sorts of things hidden in the picture, and it was a useful distraction and helped pass the time. Why can't this be in all of them? Or perhaps some poetry or something to read could help!

ACKNOWLEDGEMENTS

Bear with me – there are lots of these!

I do not even know how to express my thanks to all the healthcare professionals who have been involved in my care over nearly two years. They will never be truly able to know how deep my gratitude runs. I have put initials of those professionals who could be identified throughout the book to preserve their anonymity. Those who are named are not mentioned in the diary itself.

To Mr S–J, gynaecologist who took care and time to be thorough enough to encourage me to see a bowel surgeon, and therefore ensured that my cancer was found at an early enough stage to be treatable. To Mr N, surgeon extraordinaire, whose confidence was exactly what I needed, who answered my calls, who reassured me, who removed my cancer. To Mr M, colorectal surgeon, who managed to make me feel safe in the middle of a pandemic; Mr E, colorectal surgeon, for his care; urologist Mr G, who protected his kidney, and the wonderful anaesthetists Dr S and Dr N, who kept me sleeping and safe throughout. To Professor H, oncologist, with his calm and studied manner, who looked after me during chemotherapy and beyond. To Jacqueline Peck, colorectal cancer nurse specialist, and all the nurses and healthcare professionals involved in the hospital and clinic. To the physios, in particular Rebecca Sellars, scar management physio, who made me stand up, and helped make me pain-free, and generally encouraged me along, over many, many sessions, and who comforted me in hospital when no one else was allowed to see me.

Not forgetting the porters, cleaners, cooks and more – a hospital runs on its people, and everyone plays an essential part in that team. Special mention to the staff who often get forgotten, but ensure that doctors can do their jobs! Their secretaries and admin team, in particular Alexandra Williams, Rashika Halai and Alanna Blauch for going above and beyond, answering emails, arranging appointments and more. To my therapist, Ms D, who let me rail and cry and shout and just feel – you helped more than you could know. To all those involved with Chai Cancer Care: Graham and Johnny the physios, Jo, Debra, Samantha, Marion, Debbie and many more, who offer true holistic care to those in need. I am sure I have left people out – apologies, I am grateful to you all.

To my community of family and friends, who held us up in so many, many different ways. To those who nodded across the playground, who patted me on the back as they passed in the street, who offered help, who gave help without waiting to be asked, who rang, who left messages, who prayed for me, who showed in a myriad of ways that they were there for us. To my online support groups, in particular a private doctors' support group, which I cannot mention but they know who they are, who knew what I needed even when I didn't. To my oldest friends, Lucie, Kate and in particular my dearest friend Vicki, who were constantly in my pocket, at the end of the phone and so, so much more. Vicki, that you were able to listen and listen and listen held me up, quite literally, many, many times. And to my family, my parents, my siblings, aunts, uncles, cousins, in-laws and, most importantly, my husband and children, without you this would not have been bearable. My husband

Ben held it together at home, meaning that I could fall apart if required – oh, and he took most of the super-flattering "ill in hospital" pictures too! Words will never be enough to thank you.

To my agent, Jane Graham Maw of Graham Maw Christie Literary Agency, who was one of the first people to know as I had a book deadline shortly after my surgery (which I made!). We have now been working together for over a decade; she saw my potential a long time ago and I am so glad that our working relationship continues. To Summersdale Publishers: Clare Plimmer for believing in the work, Sophie Martin and Debbie Chapman for their editorial skills (and being kind for this one – it was hard to keep re-reading it!), Madeleine Stevens my copy-editor, who went through the manuscript with her fine-tooth comb, Jasmin Burkitt for handling all the publicity and everyone else on the Summersdale team. Thank you for handling my thoughts in this diary so gently.

◆

To the one in two of us who will get cancer at some point in our lives, and the other one in two who support those with the diagnosis, I want to say this. Thank you, for your support, in real life, online, from afar. We may go through cancer by ourselves, but we are not alone, for we have each other.

Read on for an extract from The M Word:
Everything You Need to Know About the Menopause

*Dr Kaye is the mate who's always got your back,
she knows her stuff and tells you exactly how it is.*
Sara Cox

THE

m

WORD

*Everything You Need to
Know About the Menopause*

DR PHILIPPA KAYE

FOREWORD BY VANESSA FELTZ

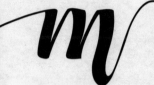

Part One:

All About the Menopause

CHAPTER 1:

BACK TO SCHOOL

◆

Brace yourselves, here comes the science bit…

If the mention of the word "science" makes you break out in a sweat, reminding you of time spent on a stool in a high-school lab, don't worry: I am going to make this as simple as possible, so please don't just skip over this section! If you have some understanding of what is going on with your hormones around the time of the menopause, then you will be able to understand better the potential treatments and choose which ones you think may suit you. Knowledge is power! So scrape your hair back, pull on an imaginary white coat (or your school uniform) and let's enter the world of your hormones.

IT'S ALL ABOUT HORMONES

The word "menopause" literally means "the last period". See, that was easy! However, we can't say that you have gone through the menopause until you haven't had a period for a year. The word for your first period is menarche, but the whole process of puberty – from growing breasts, hair and upwards to starting your periods – takes years, and so too does the period of change around the time of the menopause, called the perimenopause or climacteric.

Puberty is associated with lots of hormonal changes. The brain starts secreting a hormone called gonadotrophin-releasing hormone (GnRH), which then triggers another part of the brain to produce two further hormones, luteinising hormone (LH) and follicle-stimulating hormone (FSH). The hormones work together to trigger the ovaries to produce oestrogen, progesterone and a small amount of testosterone, and these five hormones working together cause the changes of puberty.

Once your periods (your menstrual cycle) have started, multiple hormones from the brain and ovaries work together to keep your periods coming every month. Your ovaries are found in your pelvis, on either side of the womb, and are generally about the size of an egg – a chicken's egg, that is, not a goose egg or even a human one! So here we go, high school biology coming up…

Day 1 of your menstrual cycle is day one of your period and we are going to start there. Even as you are menstruating, the part of your brain called the hypothalamus is already starting the next cycle by releasing GnRH. This in turn triggers another part of the brain, called the pituitary gland, to release follicle-stimulating hormone (FSH). Even though it is produced in the brain, FSH acts on the ovary and stimulates the development of one or more of the immature, undeveloped follicles (fluid-filled sacs which each contain an egg) in the ovary.

Still with me? Jolly good. So, the developing follicle gets bigger and the egg in it also grows and develops. Now, the cells around this follicle produce oestrogen, which has many effects in the body, but for the purposes of the menstrual cycle it acts on the lining of the womb, building it up gradually, so that if conception occurs, and a sperm has fertilized an egg, there is a nice thick lining for the egg to implant into.

So far, so good. The first half of your menstrual cycle is generally when you feel your best as a result of the rising oestrogen. The FSH and oestrogen levels gradually keep rising, and if you have a regular 28-day cycle, at about day 12–13 the pituitary gland in your brain responds to this rise by releasing a second hormone – luteinising hormone (LH). This surge triggers ovulation and the mature egg pops out of the follicle. The length of this first, follicle phase decides the length of your menstrual cycle. Once ovulation occurs, your period will start in about 14 days. So if your cycle is 28 days you will ovulate at about day 14, if it is 33 days you will ovulate at about day 19.

We're not done quite yet. Now we have an egg but the shell of the follicle from which it emerged still has work to do. It is now called the corpus luteum and produces the hormone progesterone, which again has multiple effects in the body, but in the womb acts to mature that womb lining to ensure the best conditions for egg implantation.

Almost there, no falling asleep at the back! You will still be producing some oestrogen at this point and the oestrogen and progesterone work together to maintain that all-important lining for about a further week. But unless you conceive (and this is a book about menopause and perimenopause so I am going to assume this is not what we are after) the levels of both oestrogen and progesterone fall. This means that the lining of the womb becomes unstable and is shed, and voila – you have your period.

And then the whole lot starts again over and over, month on month, until you are pregnant, or get to the point of reading this book, which is when changes are beginning to happen again.

One more hormone to mention: testosterone. It is produced by the ovaries in much smaller amounts than is produced by the testes in men, but it is there and is important, especially for your libido, or sex drive.

EGGS COUNT

Men have the capacity to continue making sperm their entire lives; they can make women pregnant from puberty right until the end of life. But women have a finite number of eggs, already predetermined before the moment they are conceived and already reduced by the time they are born, though these initial eggs that you have when you are born and as a child are very premature. Although you have many, many more eggs than you will ever need – about 1–2 million or so – about 10,000 eggs die every month until you hit puberty and by the time you get there you have about 300,000–400,000 eggs left (though the thought of 400,000 children is enough to give most of us a bit of a turn!). From the moment when you start your periods onwards you lose about 1,000 eggs a month: not all of these develop and are released, the majority get reabsorbed. Only one (sometimes two to make twins) is released each month. Only about 500 follicles mature to release an egg, so if you have a period once a month that would give you about 40 years or so of regularly having periods.

Essentially, over time, the reserves of eggs in the ovaries are depleted, and this combined with the fact that the body selects the healthiest eggs earlier in life to ovulate, means that as you get older it is harder to become pregnant. A woman's fertility starts to decline quite rapidly after the age of 35. By societal standards this is still relatively young, but reproductively it isn't!

As the number of follicles in the ovaries that can produce and release eggs continues to fall around the time of the menopause, the oestrogen and progesterone levels also begin to fall. Now, the body responds to this by whacking up how much luteinising hormone (LH) and follicle-stimulating hormone (FSH) it produces, trying harder and harder to make the ovaries produce eggs. Due to the lower levels of oestrogen and progesterone the lining of the womb doesn't build up so the periods may become irregular, further apart or even closer together until they eventually stop appearing at all.

Although 1–2 million eggs going down to virtually none may sound catastrophic, it is a natural and expected process in the body. However, for some women the menopause is brought on early, for example if they have had their ovaries removed surgically to treat cancer, or if the ovaries stop working due to chemotherapy, radiotherapy or other medications. The symptoms are the same whether or not the process was brought on by an operation or medication, or if it occurred naturally (see Chapter 3 for more detailed information about premature menopause).

After the menopause your ovaries will still produce some oestrogen, though far less than before, and some testosterone. Postmenopausal levels of progesterone are undetectable. Fat cells in the body are also capable of producing oestrogen, though in a less potent by (the chemical term is oestrone which is produced from fat cells, compared to oestradiol which is more potent and produced by the ovaries), and the adrenal glands can also produce small amounts of testosterone. So you will still naturally be producing some hormones, though at a far lower level than previously.

And relax – all done. You all get an A★, or a level 9, or whatever they are using to grade exams at the moment. (Except you in the third row who gagged at the word ovary.) Later on, when you are reading about a diet rich in phytoestrogens, and about herbs, or about hormonal medications, pop back here if you need to remind yourself of the whys and hows as this may help you decide which treatments to try.

THE PERIMENOPAUSE

Think back to puberty. That whole process took quite a few years and so do the changes relating to the menopause. Teenagers are known for being "hormonal", and puberty is associated with huge psychological, mental and emotional changes. These changes are not just around the change in their bodies but also about their change in self, as they create and develop their own personalities and behaviours with increasing independence from their parents. The menopause and perimenopause also involve an enormous amount of hormonal and physical changes and yet we seem to be kinder and more understanding towards our teenagers (even our own children) than we, or society, is to ourselves when going through the menopause. The sex hormones oestrogen, progesterone and testosterone don't just act in the genitals, ovaries and womb, they act all over the body, from the breasts to the skin. If the sex hormones act everywhere, then it is understandable that the change in levels of these hormones can have wide-ranging signs and symptoms.

As mentioned above, from as early as your late 30s and early 40s, the ovaries start not to work as effectively as before. Interestingly, many women notice that their menstrual cycle gets slightly shorter by a few days, but this doesn't mean that the menopause is imminent. This period (sorry!) can last a decade or so and in it you may get symptoms which are attributable to the menopause, from changes to your periods to flushes and sweats and mood changes. And the decline in ovarian function isn't linear; they don't gradually stop working a little less each month. Instead they can work well one month and then not the next. This also means that your hormone levels, and therefore your symptoms, can fluctuate wildly too. But fear not! Even if you are having periods – regular, irregular or totally haywire – there are still treatments that can help control your symptoms.

WHY DO WE GO THROUGH THE MENOPAUSE?

I can explain the science of what is happening at the time of the menopause, the change in your hormones and ovaries, and so on, but the purpose of the menopause is much harder to decipher. To put it in terms of an existential crisis, what is the point of it all? From an evolutionary point of view it is even harder to explain: if the point of life is to reproduce and pass on your genes, why continue to survive when you can no longer do so? And remember that this point where you may not be able to reproduce isn't even just after the menopause; in the years leading up to it your fertility declines rapidly. You can still be having periods, irregularly or regularly, but not be able to get pregnant in the years before the menopause (though for some it is still possible).

Interestingly, most mammals don't go through the menopause like we do. In general they are able to keep reproducing in older age, albeit at a reduced rate. In mammals that don't go through the menopause the chances of reproductive success decrease with age. Many fish, birds and invertebrates seem to go through a menopause – by that I am not saying their periods stop, as they don't have periods in the first place. They enter a post-reproductive stage in their lives, but they seem to die shortly afterwards. In fact, our closest genetic relatives – primates such as chimps – stop having babies in their late 30s and tend to die within a few years. Which is rather depressing. Yet human females live approximately one third of their lives after the menopause. And this isn't just in affluent countries.

So who is with us, going through the menopause and then living a substantial part of their lives afterwards? Other mammals who go through the menopause include two types of whales: the short-finned pilot whale and the killer whale.

The latter generally goes through the menopause at about 40 years old, but they can live into their 90s.

So here we are, us and the killer whales, going through the menopause. A commonly held theory as to why this occurs is the "grandmother hypothesis", which holds that older women stop reproducing so they can help with rearing their children and grandchildren, thus ensuring the survival of their children and grandchildren and thereby their own genes. Even the whales appear to do grandparent childcare! But grandmothering and the menopause don't always occur together; for example, the family structure is hugely important in elephant communities, with the matriarchs playing a significant role, and yet they don't go through the menopause. And from a maths perspective, it doesn't add up – your own children are 50% genetically yours, but your grandchildren have only 25% of your genes, so wouldn't you want those with more of your genes to survive? I am of course taking emotion out of the equation!

Another reason may be competition for resources; after all, without food no one survives. If females of all ages are competing for food as they are reproducing and focusing solely on their own children, there would be less for all. From a human point of view, if both you and your daughter are having a baby at the same time and are competing for food, the chances of survival and therefore the survival of your genes decreases. And if you add to that the higher risks of miscarriage, foetal abnormality and complications during pregnancy and labour the older you (and therefore your eggs) become, perhaps, from an evolutionary standpoint, you are better off caring for the children you already have than trying to make more. Consider how families used to work (and in some areas still do): the sons would stay in the family group but the daughters would leave and join the husband's family, to whom they generally would have no genetic connection. Therefore a daughter would gain nothing (in purely genetic terms) by helping her own mother-in-law reproduce. But once she has children and grandchildren, she has now become genetically connected to her husband's side, perhaps increasing her desire to help them survive.

Or is it simply an effect of us living longer and that some bits wear out faster than others? Hundreds of years ago we simply wouldn't have lived particularly long after the menopause. Or is it a fluke and there is no particular evolutionary logic, grand meaning or reasoning behind it at all?

I can't answer what the point of it all is – no one can – in life, as well as in the menopause. But that doesn't mean that your life doesn't have a value, purpose or point after the menopause – you can now make your own!

SUMMARY POINTS

◆ Menarche – the first period.

◆ Menopause – the last period.

◆ Climacteric – the time leading up to the last period, when hormone levels can go up and down, and the fluctuating levels can cause menopausal symptoms though you can still be having regular (or irregular) periods.

◆ Perimenopause – the time from the start of any menopausal symptoms (in the climacteric), all the way to the postmenopausal. Often though the terms climacteric and perimenopause are used interchangeably. We will use the term perimenopause throughout this book.

◆ Postmenopause – literally means "after the menopause". The menopause is a diagnosis of retrospect, in that we only say you are postmenopausal when you have not had a period for over one year. Alternatively, if you have had your ovaries removed there is no need to wait for 12 months as you will immediately be postmenopausal.

◆ The symptoms of the perimenopause and menopause are related to the change in hormone levels as the ovaries gradually stop producing eggs each month.

Have you enjoyed this book?

If so, why not write a review on your favourite website?
If you're interested in finding out more about our books,
find us on Facebook at **Summersdale Publishers**
and follow us on Twitter at **@Summersdale**.

Thanks very much for buying this Summersdale book.

www.summersdale.com